Forensic Ecology Handbook

Forensic Ecology Handbook

From Crime Scene to Court

Edited by

Nicholas Márquez-Grant

Cellmark Forensic Services, Abingdon, UK and Institute of Human Sciences, School of Anthropology and Museum of Ethnography, University of Oxford, Oxford, UK

and

Julie Roberts

Cellmark Forensic Services, Chorley, UK

WILEY-BLACKWELL

A John Wiley & Sons, Ltd., Publication

This edition first published 2012 © 2012 by John Wiley & Sons, Ltd

Wiley-Blackwell is an imprint of John Wiley & Sons, formed by the merger of Wiley's global Scientific, Technical and Medical business with Blackwell Publishing.

Registered office: John Wiley & Sons, Ltd, The Atrium, Southern Gate, Chichester, West Sussex, PO19 8SQ, UK

Editorial offices: 9600 Garsington Road, Oxford, OX4 2DQ, UK
The Atrium, Southern Gate, Chichester, West Sussex, PO19 8SQ, UK
111 River Street, Hoboken, NJ 07030-5774, USA

For details of our global editorial offices, for customer services and for information about how to apply for permission to reuse the copyright material in this book please see our website at www.wiley.com/wiley-blackwell.

The right of the author to be identified as the author of this work has been asserted in accordance with the UK Copyright, Designs and Patents Act 1988.

Library of Congress Cataloging-in-Publication Data

Forensic ecology handbook : from crime scene to court / edited by Nicholas Márquez-Grant and Julie Roberts.
    p. cm.
  Includes bibliographical references and index.
  ISBN 978-1-119-97419-2 (cloth)
  1. Forensic sciences.   2. Forensic anthropology.   3. Forensic archaeology.   4. Forensic botany.
5. Environmental sciences.   6. Crime scene investigation.   I. Márquez-Grant, Nicholas, 1976-
II. Roberts, Julie (Julie J.)
  HV8073.F564 2012
  363.25–dc23

                                                                                      2012016770

A catalogue record for this book is available from the British Library.

Wiley also publishes its books in a variety of electronic formats. Some content that appears in print may not be available in electronic books.

Set in 10.5/12.5pt Times by Aptara Inc., New Delhi, India.

First Impression   2012

Contents

About the Editors

Dr Nicholas Márquez-Grant is a Forensic Anthropologist and Archaeologist at Cellmark Forensic Services (UK), having worked previously for other forensic science providers and commercial archaeological units. He is also a Research Associate of the Institute of Human Sciences, School of Anthropology and Museum Ethnography, University of Oxford. Having worked as a specialist in human skeletal remains from archaeological sites for over 15 years, he has considerable experience in the excavation and study of cremated and unburnt bone from prehistoric sites to twentieth-century conflict sites and from a variety of geographical areas in Europe, and in particular Spain. Dr Márquez-Grant has taught biological anthropology since 2001 at the University of Oxford where he was awarded his doctoral degree in archaeology and physical anthropology in 2006. In recent years he has worked full-time as a forensic anthropologist and archaeologist in cases from a large number of police forces in the United Kingdom, dealing with the search, recovery, location and identification of human remains, and has acted as an expert witness. He also trains crime scene investigators from a number of forces in the United Kingdom and abroad.

Dr Julie Roberts is Scientific Lead and Team Leader for the Anthropology, Archaeology and Ecology Department at Cellmark Forensic Services (UK). She is a biological anthropologist and archaeologist by background with over 15 years' experience working in archaeology and at crime scenes, excavating and examining decomposed, skeletonised, fragmented, burnt and commingled human remains. Her forensic experience includes deployment as forensic anthropologist with the British Forensic Team in Kosovo in 1999, 2000 and 2002, exhumation and examination of murder victims in Iraq in 2003, and lead anthropologist following the London bombings in 2005 and the Nimrod air crash in 2006. Recent casework includes successfully locating, recovering and assisting in the identification of human remains in Lebanon and mass fatality deployments to Afghanistan. Dr Roberts has attended numerous crime scenes of different types across the United Kingdom, specialising in the excavation and analysis of burnt and fragmented remains. She is one of only two forensic anthropologists who sit in the expert panel for UK Disaster Victim Identification. She is registered with the National Policing Improvement Agency (NPIA) as an expert advisor in anthropology and archaeology, and has been involved in instructing police officers and crime scene investigators for over 10 years.

List of Contributors

Beverley Adams-Groom, National Pollen and Aerobiology Unit (NPARU), University of Worcester, Worcester, UK

Sophie Beckett, Cranfield Forensic Institute, Cranfield University, Shrivenham, UK

Ruth Buckley, Metropolitan Police Service, London, UK

Gordon Cook, Scottish Universities Environmental Research Group (SUERC), East Kilbride, Scotland, UK

Eileen J. Cox, Natural History Museum, London, UK

Martin Hall, Department of Life Sciences, Natural History Museum, London, UK

Andy Langley, Metropolitan Police Service, London, UK

Stephen Litherland, Cellmark Forensic Services, Abingdon, UK

Nicholas Márquez-Grant, Cellmark Forensic Services, Abingdon, UK; and Institute of Human Sciences, School of Anthropology and Museum Ethnography, University of Oxford, Oxford, UK

Peter Massey, Forensic Science Department, Henry C. Lee College of Criminal Justice and Forensic Sciences, University of New Haven, West Haven, CT, USA

Andrew McDonald, Cellmark Forensic Services, Abingdon, UK

Heather Miller Coyle, Forensic Science Department, Henry C. Lee College of Criminal Justice and Forensic Sciences, University of New Haven, West Haven, CT, USA

Duncan Pirrie, Helford Geoscience LLP, Penryn, UK

Cameron Richards, Department of Life Sciences, Natural History Museum, London, UK

Julie Roberts, Cellmark Forensic Services, Chorley, UK

Alastair Ruffell, School of Geography, Archaeology and Palaeoecology, Queen's University Belfast, Belfast, Northern Ireland, UK

Peter Valentin, Forensic Science Department, Henry C. Lee College of Criminal Justice and Forensic Sciences, University of New Haven, West Haven, CT, USA

Mark Viner, Inforce Foundation, Cranfield Forensic Institute, Shrivenham, UK; and St Bartholomew's and The Royal London Hospitals, London, UK

Michael Walbank, Cellmark Forensic Services, Abingdon, UK

Chris Webster, Cheshire Constabulary, Cheshire, UK

Amoret Whitaker, Department of Life Sciences, Natural History Museum, London, UK

John Yoward, Cellmark Forensic Services, Abingdon, UK

Series Foreword
Developments in forensic science

In the past few years the development of teaching, research and knowledge exchange activities associated with forensic science policy and practice have increased almost exponentially. Technological innovations, the pursuit of new knowledge and the interpretation of analytical and other data as it is applied within forensic practice is to be welcomed as we move to a phase where our profession is striving towards gaining a foothold on maturity as a science. Practising forensic scientists are constantly striving to deliver the very best in their service to the judicial process and as such need a reliable and robust knowledge base within their diverse disciplines.

As we develop new knowledge and address the research and practical application issues within the field, the consolidation and dissemination of new methdodologies relevant to forensic science practice becomes essential. It is the objective of this book series to provide a valuable resource for forensic science practitioners, educators and others in that regard. The books developed and published within this series come from some of the leading researchers and practitioners in their fields and will provide essential and relevant information to the reader.

Professor Niamh Nic Daéid
Series Editor

Foreword

Jonathan Smith
National Forensic Specialist Adviser
National Policing Improvement Agency, UK

Traditionally forensic science has been organised in terms of the scientific disciplines, for example biology, chemistry, drugs and toxicology, and firearms.

The scientists involved in the examination of casework exhibits in many instances have extended their expertise across the disciplines giving a more integrated view of the sciences that can be applied to the varying situations appearing in police investigations.

Taking the biology specialism of forensic science as an example, this has mostly dealt with the wide range of biological materials that might be transferred during the commission of a crime. This could be the transfer of blood and body fluids, hair, textile fibres and botanical material. It is fair to say that the examination of transferred botanical material has in the past not really featured as a major consideration in many investigations.

Over the last decade there is no doubt that the focus of the science applied to forensic science cases has centred on developments in DNA technologies. Some of the other scientific skills applied to forensic science have to a large extent been less well supported. This situation at one stage led to the development of sciences such as botany, entomology, archaeology and anthropology being centred on academic institutes, or in some instances experts acting alone.

Consequently this resulted in an almost peripheral group of experts, who were seen as detached from mainstream forensic science, confined by the boundaries of their discipline, and who relied upon their individual reputation rather than a corporate assurance implied by the traditional forensic science providers.

The situation now is distinctly different, with a greater integration of these specialist disciplines into forensic science.

In this volume the expertise in these various disciplines is brought together for the use of investigators, specialists and those working within the criminal justice system. The structures that are in place within a major crime investigation, and the roles and responsibilities of the investigation team are outlined, and there is an explanation of how the various elements of the team interact. Also included in the text is some specific detail for the practitioner outlining sampling procedures, packaging and exhibit examination practices.

There is recognition by the contributors of the ultimate responsibility of the expert to present to the court the scientific findings in a balanced manner, mindful of the need for quality, peer review and an assurance that the science being applied is based on published data and tested principles. In this way the confidence in the application of these scientific disciplines into an all-encompassing forensic science response to crime investigation is greatly enhanced.

Foreword

Richard T. Shepherd
Consultant Forensic Pathologist, UK

One of the many changes that has occurred during the 30 years that I have been practising forensic pathology is the rise of forensic science. To cite but one example, blood serology, which relied upon the visual identification of antibody agglutination of red blood cells which determine the major and minor blood groups present, has been swept away by DNA analysis. This has resulted in an increase in the specificity and accuracy of blood analysis by a factor of many millions. However, this apparent 'certainty' has meant that if there was a mistake it would in all probability be a big one. Instead of the accepted 'possible error' of blood serology, DNA resulted in statements approximating to certainty which may have reflected the science but they did not allow for fundamentally faulty practice.

And there were setbacks when enthusiasm exceeded reliable, scientific analysis and sound forensic practice. When those results and opinions were robustly tested by other practitioners in the laboratory and then by the lawyers in the courts, parts were exposed to be flawed and the whole edifice collapsed. These moments are salutary lessons for us all, for they inform us that just because we think that something might be right that does not in itself make it right. We must build our skills and our expertise and our evidence on the solid foundations of knowledge, experience and adherence to strict forensic practices.

The process of scene examination has also progressed in ways that simply could not have been anticipated in the 1980s. At one time, the forensic pathologist did just about everything at the scene – seldom even wearing overshoes – and now everyone wears full protective clothing and the pathologist gets to do very little indeed because they no longer have the full set of skills that are needed, but they have to be aware of the whole spectrum of specialist skills and experience that the forensic scientists can bring to a scene or a post-mortem examination.

As the apparent accuracy of forensic science increases, the subject in all its many forms is becoming increasingly important in this modern, litigatious world. The interface between science and the law, whether civil or criminal, is becoming more challenging and it is essential that there are forensic science practitioners available to the police, to the defence and above all to the courts. Those practitioners must have the requisite knowledge, skills, and also the experience to perform the highly complex, specialist scene and laboratory examinations in a forensically satisfactory manner. They must also be able to produce and give reliable, science-based evidence that will enable the court to reach their verdict with a full understanding of the facts and confidence in their source.

Despite the longevity of forensic science as a whole, the subject continues to develop new specialist areas in response to scientific advances combined with pressure from the police and the criminal justice system. The over-arching speciality of Forensic Ecology that is the subject of this book covers both the well-established fields of archaeology and anthropology and also extends into rather more recently developed fields such as forensic botany.

This textbook emphasises the need for a methodical, careful and precise approach to all problems. It accepts that not all practitioners will have all of the precise skills that may eventually be needed in any particular case and it emphasises that the adoption of the correct approach will allow others – possibly someone with greater specialist skills or maybe just the expert acting for the defence – to understand and to rely on the processes by which the information was obtained so that opinions will be based on reliably obtained evidence.

Those who choose to practise forensic science must now move their subjects forward. They must ensure that current and future practitioners are both skilled and experienced in all the relevant areas of practice and they must ensure that the police, the courts and the public insist on that professionalism and expertise. The authors have ensured that this present volume is specifically designed to be practical and they have included useful, focused and reliable advice on the handling of casework throughout the text. The case histories that are also included provide a superb basis for learning and for the understanding of both basic and more advanced forensic concepts. However the practice of forensic medicine does not stop at the examination of a scene or the examination of the victim or perpetrator and this handbook recognises these crucial aspects and also deals with the task of report writing and the giving of evidence in court.

This excellent volume is a thorough and complete overview of this speciality and provides a reliable and comprehensive textbook that is suitable both for practitioners already working within this field and for those seeking to develop a specialist interest and skill in Forensic Ecology. Julie Roberts and Nicholas Márquez-Grant have extensive knowledge and skill and have worked for many years in their own fields. To bring to one book such experience and expertise is rare and their joint efforts in producing this book reflects their immense knowledge and enthusiasm for their subject.

1

Introduction

Nicholas Márquez-Grant[1] and Julie Roberts[2]
[1]Cellmark Forensic Services, Abingdon, UK; and Institute of Human Sciences, School of Anthropology and Museum Ethnography, University of Oxford, Oxford, UK
[2]Cellmark Forensic Services, Chorley, UK

This volume stems from the editors' experience in archaeology and anthropology as applied to criminal investigation. Archaeologists have always been familiar with sampling for soils, pollen and other environmental sources to provide information about ancient landscapes and for their contribution to our understanding of the past. Likewise, physical anthropologists specialising in human skeletal anatomy have studied demographic profiles, disease patterns and funerary practices in past societies with the purpose of understanding the lifestyles and environment of pre-modern populations.

The disciplines of archaeology and anthropology (whether under the same umbrella or as separate fields of study), are closely interlinked with environmental sciences such as palynology, botany, pedology, geology and entomology. This applies in both modern and ancient contexts, although the way in which they are used will vary according to the questions being asked. For example, the physical anthropologist and palynologist working on an Iron Age settlement site might be utilising their skills to assess the life expectancy, health, diet and nutritional status of the people who once lived there, whereas at a crime scene the same expertise might be used to establish the identity of the deceased and to link a suspect to a scene. In both cases, the science and the principles behind it remain the same, although the specialists engaged in forensic casework need to have a good working knowledge of the criminal justice system of the country they are working in, and an awareness of their place within it.

The anthropologist or archaeologist dealing with human remains of forensic or medico-legal interest, should be familiar, prior to recovery of the remains, with a wide range of other forensic disciplines. This includes a general awareness of biomolecular and biological trace evidence and body fluids such as DNA, saliva, blood and semen, as well as other forensic evidence types including fibres, fingerprints and footwear marks. They should have a more detailed knowledge of pollen,

Forensic Ecology Handbook: From Crime Scene to Court, First Edition.
Edited by Nicholas Márquez-Grant and Julie Roberts.
© 2012 John Wiley & Sons, Ltd. Published 2012 by John Wiley & Sons, Ltd.

plants, diatoms and insects, which in our experience can often provide vital information relating to post-mortem interval (time-since-death), the manner in which the victim was disposed of, seasonality and even cause of death.

Whilst environmental evidence requires the attention of highly specialised scientists it is important that the anthropologist or archaeologist, who will often take the scientific lead on complex cases where remains are extensively decomposed, has a good appreciation of the potential applications of the related scientific techniques. It is also vital that they are trained and experienced in the collection of pollen, soil, insect and plant specimens in case the appropriate specialist is unable to attend the scene (although attendance by the appropriate specialist is always recommended as best practice).

Conversely it is important that police and crime scene investigators understand the role of the archaeologist, anthropologist and environmental scientist at the crime scene and how their specific areas of expertise can benefit a criminal investigation.

The disciplines of archaeology, anthropology, palynology, botany and entomology among others, can be used together to assist in the search, location, recovery and identification of human remains (and other buried evidence such as firearms or drugs). They can be utilised to indicate how much time has passed since the body was left at the scene and link suspects to scenes and victims, and they can be used to answer specific questions such as: Who is the victim? How long has the victim been dead? Is there a third party involved? How long has the victim been at a particular deposition or burial site? How did he or she die? And what happened after the death of the individual, for example did the suspect re-visit the scene, did animals damage the remains, or was the body moved? It should also be noted that the work of these specialists is not restricted to outdoor scenes and anthropologists and entomologists in particular may frequently be required to attend deaths in houses, garages or other indoor locations.

In this volume we encompass the environmental sciences within the term 'Forensic Ecology'. This is a broad description and its use can be extended to areas such as wildlife and environmental crime incorporating a wide range of applications. However, in this book we restrict ourselves largely to major crime, focusing on how anthropology, archaeology and ecology can aid in the investigation of missing persons, suspicious and unexplained deaths.

Many books have been published on the individual subjects of forensic anthropology, forensic archaeology, forensic entomology, forensic botany or forensic geology (e.g. Hunter and Cox, 2005; Blau and Ubelaker, 2009; Schmitt, Cunha and Pinheiro, 2006; Komar and Buikstra, 2008; Byrd and Castner, 2009; Gennard, 2007; Miller Coyle, 2005; Ruffell and McKinley, 2008). These volumes provide an introduction to each discipline, background information on the science, provide case studies and explain the methods involved, as do many of the thousands of scientific papers that have been published throughout the years. There are also volumes that include these areas of expertise in general introductory texts to forensic science or criminalistics (e.g. Saferstein, 2011; White, 2004; Anadón and Robledo, 2010; Gunn, 2006; James and Nordby, 2005). This book, however, focuses on drawing together disciplines specifically related to environmental sciences, victim recovery and identification. It is aimed at forensic science practitioners and police officers currently involved in crime scene investigation as well as those still studying or working as trainees. It will provide them with an awareness of the potential applications of these disciplines and hopefully give them the confidence to decide when to call out the appropriate specialist and how to best preserve the evidence at the scene until they get there. The practical information relating to collection of ecological samples will ensure that police officers and crime scene investigators are in the best position to ensure that good practice is being utilised by the specialist they have invited to the scene. They may also have to follow the guidelines themselves in emergency situations where, for example, there is a long delay before the scientist can attend, the scene is remote or cannot be secured for any length of time. Forensic ecology is a discipline rarely taught in standard police or crime scene investigator training and as such this book can fill a potentially wide knowledge gap.

In addition to focusing on environmental evidence types, victim recovery and identification, we have set out to clarify aspects of crime scene management and police procedures which relate directly to the specialist at the scene. The importance of continuity and integrity of evidence is reiterated in a number of chapters throughout the book as it is vital for the practitioner to understand that whilst their specialist knowledge, expertise and results might be first class, if they fail to follow proper procedure (for example failing to sign an exhibit label or seal an item at the scene) their evidence may be rendered inadmissible with potentially disastrous results for a case. This was illustrated in the recent re-trial of two men accused of the murder of Stephen Lawrence in South London in 1993 (Daily Mail, 2012). The case for the prosecution almost fell apart not because of flaws in the scientific analysis and findings, but because some of the evidence had been stored in exhibit bags that had not been sealed, thereby providing the defence with an ideal opportunity to allege that the forensic evidence was in fact contamination which had occurred after the event.

The contributors in this book are extremely experienced forensic practitioners with a wealth of knowledge. The volume is structured in a way that provides a useful guide to forensic scientists and practitioners about the evidence types involved in the recovery and identification of human remains from forensic contexts.

Each chapter provides background information on the discipline it is concerned with and is structured in a logical sequence progressing through preparation prior to attending a scene (What questions should the scientist ask when receiving a call from a police force? What equipment do they need to prepare before attending a scene?), the scene attendance itself (including protocols at the scene, sampling strategies, recording), scientific examination and analysis of the evidence in the laboratory, and finally the production of an expert witness statement and court testimony.

In Chapter 2, aspects of crime scene management written by Forensic Practitioners from the Metropolitan Police Service in London are discussed. This relates primarily to roles and procedures employed in England and Wales, but the key personnel involved in crime scene investigation and the principles adhered to at the scene are standard in most developed countries. Chapter 3 deals with forensic archaeology. This volume perceives archaeology and anthropology to be separate, albeit inter-related, disciplines, although in some countries archaeology may be seen as a subdiscipline of anthropology. Chapter 4 describes the role of the anthropologist in victim identification and in the assessment of post-mortem interval. It also summarises how the anthropologist's knowledge of skeletal anatomy can assist the pathologist in determining cause of death by physical reconstruction of remains and trauma analysis. It is followed by chapters on the use of radiography (Chapter 5) and sampling for DNA (Chapter 6) in victim identification. Other techniques that might be of assistance in determining post-mortem interval or the identity of the deceased include radiocarbon dating and isotope analysis (Chapter 7). Entomology is covered in Chapter 8, primarily with the aim of inferring post-mortem interval, whilst Chapters 9 to 12 deal with other ecological evidence types: diatoms, palynology, botany and geology. Chapter 13 provides an in-depth discussion on Police Exhibits including clear guidelines on what constitutes an exhibit, how to produce, label, document and store them. It also provides vital information relating to avoidance of the pitfalls that can so easily beset the practitioner if the correct procedures are not followed. Finally, Forensic Photography is a fundamental part of crime scene investigation and forms the primary record for attendance at any scene or examination. Chapter 14 describes the standard techniques used in Forensic Photography and guidelines for best practice to ensure that any images taken are relevant, include all the required information (for example a means of orientation, scale and exhibit number depending on the subject matter), and are of an acceptable standard to be presented in court.

We hope this book will be of some value to practitioners, police staff, academics and students, who may be required to attend crime scenes where human remains and ecological evidence types are present. We anticipate that it will enable them to realise the potential applications surrounding the disciplines of anthropology, archaeology and environmental science and give them a broader awareness of how a wide range of related scientific techniques can assist in victim recovery, identification and criminal investigation.

This volume would not have been possible without the tireless effort of our contributors, who we greatly thank for their time and their expertise. They are all experienced practitioners who have written their chapters whilst working full-time in their chosen fields. We are grateful for the support given by colleagues at Cellmark Forensic Services, UK, as well as friends and relatives during the process of editing this book. We would also like to express our gratitude to the staff at Wiley-Blackwell, especially Rachael Ballard and Fiona Seymour.

References

Anadón Baselga, M.J. and Robledo Acinas, M.M. (eds) 2010. *Manual de Criminalística y Ciencias Forenses. Técnicas Forenses Aplicadas a la Investigación Criminal.* Editorial Tébar S.L., Madrid.

Blau, S. and Ubelaker, D.H. (eds) 2009. *Handbook of Forensic Anthropology and Archaeology.* Left Coast Press, Walnut Creek, CA.

Byrd, J.H. and Castner, J.L. 2009. *Forensic Entomology: The Utility of Arthropods in Legal Investigations*, 2nd edn. CRC Press, Boca Raton, FL.

Daily Mail: http://www.dailymail.co.uk/news/article-2079782/Stephen-Lawrence-trial-Gary-Dobson-David-Norris-guilty-murder.html (accessed 12 January 2012).

Gennard, D.E. 2007. *Forensic Entomology: An Introduction.* John Wiley & Sons, Ltd, Chichester.

Gunn, A. 2006. *Essential Forensic Biology.* John Wiley & Sons, Ltd, Chichester.

Hunter, J. and Cox, M. 2005. *Forensic Archaeology: Advances in Theory and Practice.* Routledge, London.

James, S.H. and Nordby, J.J. (eds) 2005. *Forensic Science: An Introduction to Scientific and Investigative Techniques*, 2nd edn. CRC Press/Taylor & Francis, Boca Raton, FL.

Komar, D.A. and Buikstra, J.E. 2008. *Forensic Anthropology: Contemporary Theory and Practice.* Oxford University Press, New York.

Miller Coyle, H. (ed.) 2005. *Forensic Botany: Principles and Applications to Criminal Casework.* CRC Press, Boca Raton, FL.

Ruffell, A. and McKinley, J. 2008. *Geoforensics.* John Wiley & Sons, Ltd, Chichester.

Saferstein, R. 2011. *Criminalistics: An Introduction to Forensic Science*, 10th edn. Pearson-Prentice Hall, Upper Saddle River, NJ.

Schmitt, A., Cunha, E. and Pinheiro, J. (eds) 2006. *Forensic Anthropology and Medicine: Complementary Sciences from Recovery to Cause of Death.* Human Press Inc., Totowa, NJ.

White, P.C. (ed.). 2004. *Crime Scene to Court: The Essentials of Forensic Science*, 2nd edn. The Royal Society of Chemistry, London.

2

Aspects of crime scene management

Ruth Buckley and Andy Langley
Metropolitan Police Service, London, UK

2.1 Introduction

This chapter is divided into two parts. The first will review specific police roles and professionals working at major crime scenes such as homicide. This aims to provide the reader with an understanding of the structure and roles within an investigative team and its associated personnel. The second part of this chapter will focus on working at crime scenes from basic procedures and the employment of specialists to the conclusion of work and provision of statements. This aims to provide sufficient background and forensic awareness to enable the reader to work confidently at a crime scene in conjunction with police personnel. The experience of both authors is based on their work within the Metropolitan Police Service (MPS). Therefore it must be acknowledged that the protocols and practices to be discussed here may vary elsewhere in the United Kingdom and will be different abroad.

2.2 Professionals within the investigation

A great number of individuals are involved in the investigation of serious crime and homicide from its initial reporting through to the collation and presentation of evidence at court. It would be impractical to list every role performed and in terms of crime scene examination and management, not every position requires explanation here. The individual roles to be discussed form by no means an exhaustive list and do not seek to belittle other essential positions within an investigation by their exclusion. Therefore those selected for discussion are the most pertinent with reference to working at crime scenes, the mortuary and within the forensic examination of exhibits.

Forensic Ecology Handbook: From Crime Scene to Court, First Edition.
Edited by Nicholas Márquez-Grant and Julie Roberts.
© 2012 John Wiley & Sons, Ltd. Published 2012 by John Wiley & Sons, Ltd.

2.2.1 Senior Investigating Officer

The Senior Investigating Officer (SIO) is a complex role holding overall charge of an investigation and the accountability for the conduct of the enquiry (ACPO, 2006); this position is usually held by a Detective Chief Inspector. The SIO is responsible for the development of the investigative strategy and implementation of an effective team structure and process to manage the information coming into and produced by the investigation team (ACPO, 2006). The SIO ensures that the team is adequately staffed and with the Deputy SIO, appoints key individuals to specific roles within the enquiry (ACPO, 2005). SIOs have considerable experience and knowledge in addition to strong leadership and communication skills providing them with the ability to deal with the most complex investigations often in the media spotlight. The SIO will (with the assistance of others) manage both the media and community concerns. It is usual for a Deputy SIO to assist with managerial aspects of the enquiry, enabling the SIO to focus on the strategic aspects of the investigation (ACPO, 2006). The SIO will expect to attend a crime scene which enables them to formulate appropriate strategies and to lead the enquiry effectively. The SIO may attend post-mortems, but will usually task a Detective Inspector to attend on their behalf to brief the Forensic Pathologist and to clarify the implications of any cause of death given and findings of the pathologist.

2.2.2 The Enquiry Team

In addition to the SIO a homicide investigation team usually is comprised of three Detective Inspectors, two of whom lead core teams comprised of Detective Sergeants and Constables. The third Inspector leads the intelligence unit and the major incident room (MIR) which is comprised of Detective Sergeants and Constables and police staff fulfilling analyst, researcher and indexer roles (ACPO, 2005). The MIR runs the Home Office Large Major Enquiry System (HOLMES) which is used to manage the information within the enquiry. A number of specialist roles within the enquiry team are performed by trained officers. The role of Family Liaison Officer (FLO) is primarily investigative acting as a conduit between the family of a victim and the enquiry team providing support and information pertaining to the deceased. CCTV-trained officers identify and interrogate footage which can often yield crucial information. Members of the enquiry team may attend the crime scene as an investigation develops in order to familiarise themselves with geographic or contextual aspects of the scene and to aid their interpretation of information coming into the enquiry.

2.2.3 The Exhibits Officer

A role usually performed by a Detective Constable, the Exhibits Officer (EO) takes overall responsibility for each exhibit recovered in an investigation providing a resilient presence at crime scenes and the mortuary. Using exhibits books (see Section 2.4.3) they ensure the continuity and integrity of exhibits until all necessary legal actions are complete (ACPO, 2005; Weston, 1998) when they will then arrange for exhibits to be restored to an individual and retained by police or destroyed (ACPO, 2005; Weston, 1998).

2.2.4 Disclosure Officer

An officer will be appointed who is responsible for disclosing all the information that has been identified or produced during an enquiry to the Crown Prosecution Service (CPS) who will serve this information to the defence counsel unless it is deemed to be sensitive (ACPO, 2005).

2.2.5 Crime Scene Manager

The role of the Crime Scene Manager (CSM) is held by an individual experienced in the examination and interpretation of crime scenes with a comprehensive forensic knowledge. They possess strong leadership skills allowing them to efficiently manage scenes facilitating specialists in the best and most appropriate order to maximise the forensic potential. The role requires knowledge of many forensic disciplines and how they interact and impact upon each other, which is vital when determining the sequence of examination.

The CSM works alongside the SIO, managing the forensic input into an enquiry, attending scenes and conducting assessments and interpretations to determine appropriate examination strategies which will then be discussed and agreed with the SIO in order to jointly formulate a forensic strategy before the examination begins (ACPO, 2006). They are responsible for managing scenes, health and safety considerations and providing detailed briefings for those in attendance (Duhig and Turnbull, 2007; Hunter and Cox, 2005), coordinating the crime scene examination and the attendance of appropriate specialists and photographers (Menez, 2005). The CSM ensures that the necessary resources and logistics are available which may include stepping plates, screening, cover, lighting or other specialist equipment such as the construction of temporary structures to protect potential evidence from adverse weather (Specialist Crime Policy Unit, 2008a). In complex enquiries the CSM may delegate the management of individual scenes to other CSMs.

The CSM attends post-mortem examinations in homicide or unexplained death investigations and will ensure the forensic strategy agreed with the SIO is relayed to the forensic pathologist. The CSM maintains the forensic management of an enquiry to its conclusion, recommending, agreeing and overseeing all submissions, collating results and controlling the forensic budget of each investigation. The CSM will review forensic results against the forensic strategy, re-evaluate and consider further submissions establishing a rationale for this. They ensure a proportionate response of finite resources recognising the complexities in major crime that can require not only forensic identification, but also forensic reconstruction. The CSM also facilitates any meetings between forensic specialists and the SIO where necessary. They will often meet with counsel attending case management meetings in order to ensure that the value of the forensic evidence is fully understood. The CSMs produce statements of all their work within an investigation and give evidence at court as required.

2.2.6   Forensic Practitioner

The role of a Forensic Practitioner is often more commonly referred to as a SOCO (Scenes of Crime Officer), Forensic Investigator or Crime Scene Examiner amongst other variants. While the title may vary, the ethos of the profession is very similar: to attend crime scenes and recover forensic and fingermark evidence (Hunter and Knupfer, 1997; Pepper, 2005). In the case of homicide investigations the examiner will work under the direction of a CSM. Forensic practitioners receive extensive training in the recognition and retrieval of forensic evidence and are fully conversant with current protocols and best practice in packaging exhibits, working with the highest integrity ensuring the continuity of crime scene exhibits (Anderson *et al.*, 2008a; Hunter and Knupfer, 1997; Pepper, 2005). Forensic practitioners work in conjunction with the EO and specialists as directed by the CSM providing support and assistance where necessary (Hunter and Cox, 2005). They have broad expertise and backgrounds and this can be recognised in the range of tasks performed.

2.2.7   Forensic Photographer

The Forensic Photographer produces both video, and still images at scenes, at the mortuary and in the studio. Their role is important in recording the crime scene providing visual evidence for the enquiry team and judicial system (Fisher, 1992). It is often preferable, early on in an enquiry, to brief team members through viewing these images and videos. Photographers produce primary evidence in the photography of fingermarks and footwear marks which are technically demanding; their wide-ranging experience is highly beneficial in obtaining the best results from scenes and the mortuary alike. Thus it is important for specialists to fully brief them, highlighting areas of interest in order to capture the required images.

2.2.8   Evidence Recovery Unit

Nationally there are many different interpretations of the Evidence Recovery Unit (ERU) model as used within the MPS. They are essentially a team of forensic experts from different disciplines that deploy as a bespoke unit utilising their skills and experience in the identification and recovery of differing strands of evidence. This includes blood pattern analysis, body fluids, trace evidence, DNA and fingermarks. Within the team are specialist photographers, who are able to utilise a wide range of techniques aiding the search and recovery of evidence using specialist light sources and radiology. They possess enhanced equipment which are vital tools at complex scenes including high level cameras (Skycam) and immersive imaging (360° photography). The team also includes members skilled in the chemical enhancement and development of fingermarks.

2.2.9 Police Search Advisor Team

The Police Search Advisor team more commonly known as POLSA are a group of Police Officers led by a Police Sergeant with advanced and extensive training in search methods, techniques and the recognition of evidence (Hunter and Cox, 2005; Pepper, 2005). They work under the direction of the Investigating Officer and CSM and are often employed to search large areas and venues (ACPO, 2006; Duhig and Turnball, 2007). Officers within the team do not seize evidence they identify, this is done by the EO or forensic practitioner.

2.2.10 Home Office Pathologist

Similarly to crime scene examination the role of the Forensic Pathologist has received vast attention in television and film. One cannot discuss professionals within a homicide investigation without acknowledging their involvement. In the MPS it is not common for a pathologist to attend every crime scene to examine the body *in situ*; however, the authors acknowledge that this prevalence is different elsewhere in national and international contexts. The request for a pathologist to attend the scene is made by the CSM in agreement with the SIO (ACPO, 2006), for example in complex cases such as buried contexts (Menez, 2005) or in circumstances when recovery could inflict damage to the remains. The CSM will agree with the pathologist should any examination of the body need to take place prior to the post-mortem, for example to avoid loss of evidence.

2.2.11 The Coroner

Within England and Wales, the Coroner has absolute authority over issues relating to deceased individuals recovered in their area. Any actions around the discovery, removal and examination of human remains must only be done with the permission of the Coroner (ACPO, 2006). In practical terms, contact will usually be made via the Coroner's Officer who will make any necessary arrangements and consult with or advise the Coroner as required. In requesting permission to move a body from a scene to a mortuary the Coroner's Officer will nominate which mortuary is to be used and will secure the services of a pathologist, if one has not already been deployed (ACPO, 2006). It is not usual practice to move a body out of a Coroner's geographic jurisdiction, therefore any request to utilise a particular mortuary, perhaps if a specific examination is required, needs to be fully explained and communicated in advance.

Initial communication with the Coroner's Officer is usually made by the CSM who remains the focal point for all issues relating to the body and is responsible for updating them with any relevant facts. A Coroner's Officer may attend the scene, but access should only be granted where there is a specific purpose and there is no risk of compromising the integrity of the scene. It is usual for the Coroner's Officer to attend the post-mortem and on behalf of the Coroner they will expect to receive the names and contact details of all those in attendance as well as a record of the exhibits taken.

2.2.12　Uniformed Police Officer

All crime scenes are secured and guarded and this role is most commonly performed by a uniformed Police Officer. This is essential to ensure the security and integrity of the crime scene and maintain the crime scene log. At large scenes it is not uncommon to have multiple cordon officers rotated over shifts as crime scenes can remain open for protracted lengths of time. The cordon officer is often the focal point for those attending scenes to work in addition to members of the public and media. They are responsible for the recording of information of personnel within the crime scene and ensuring that no unauthorised individuals are permitted entry.

2.3　Crime scene principles

2.3.1　The crime scene

In simple terms a crime scene could be defined as a place where a crime has been committed (Horswell, 2004); however, this does not fully encompass the nature and reality of crime scene investigation and management. Forensic evidence is not singularly bound to a primary location where an offence took place. Essentially a crime scene is identified and created by a Police Officer with spatial parameters recognising that the area enclosed could contain information and evidence pertinent to a crime (Skinner and Sterenberg, 2005). A crime scene should not only be considered as a location or place but can also be a person such as a suspect or victim, or an object. Therefore perhaps a more comprehensive definition of a crime scene would be a place, person or object with the potential to yield forensic evidence pertaining to an investigation. This distinction is not simply academic as the recognition of separate scenes is important to ensure the integrity of evidence and to guard against contamination.

2.3.2 Security and protection

Upon the identification of a crime scene, Police Officers take further steps to secure and protect it (Fisher, 1992). This takes the form of physical barriers such as a cordon tape with Police Officers strategically placed around the perimeter to control the admission of authorised personnel (ACPO, 2006; Pepper, 2005; Specialist Crime Policy Unit, 2008a). Access and egress paths are established to minimize crime scene disturbance and a rendezvous point is agreed; concurrently a crime scene log is opened.

In addition to the security rationale, the protection of crime scenes is necessary to prevent changes occurring to forensic evidence and its later interpretation (Horswell, 2004). Everything is preserved *in situ* as originally found to preclude the movement, change, alteration and loss of forensic evidence (ACPO, 2006; Horswell, 2004; Specialist Crime Policy Unit, 2008a). Scene tents, tarpaulins and temporary structures are often implemented to this end and can be seen as synonymous with crime scene working in the media; however, they also serve to protect the scene and personnel working.

Once established, a crime scene is policed, secured and protected. What happens next is variable and determined on a case by case basis. The SIO and CSM dictate scene admittance and the work undertaken by whom and when. Every case is different and variables such as the time, weather, lighting and location can be influential in the decision-making and scene management process. All actions, initial strategies and decisions are recorded ensuring that the investigation is accountable, transparent and justified.

2.3.3 Chain of Custody

This term refers to the movement of an exhibit from its initial finding through to presentation at court (Cobb, 1998; Horswell, 2004; Pepper, 2005; Weston, 1998). It is paramount to provide a documented trail of precisely when and where an exhibit was retrieved, transported, stored, analysed and specifically who handled it (ACPO, 2006). Exhibits can be moved and examined by numerous individuals therefore it is important to fully record their journey to ensure transparency and full accountability (Fisher, 1992). Any changes to an exhibit such as division for examination must be documented and any newly created exhibits recorded. The EO's role is crucial in ensuring that the chain of custody is correctly adhered to throughout an investigation (Nicol *et al.*, 2004). Specialists working within criminal investigations must adhere to this method of working, fully documenting and logging the movement of exhibits within their place of work and similarly recording handling personnel (see Chapter 13).

2.3.4 Continuity

The term continuity is fundamental in forensic and criminal investigations referring to the proof of the chain of evidence (Weston, 1998). This corroborative support is provided by meticulous documentation, records, contemporaneous notes, scene logs and receipts (Donnelly *et al.*, 2008). On every exhibit seized there is a designated area on the label for signatures which provides verification of those seizing and handling (Horswell, 2004).

2.3.5 Integrity

In a similar way to continuity and when taken in conjunction with crime scene working and exhibits, integrity refers to working in an honest and upright manner ensuring that the scene and exhibits are protected against either deliberate or accidental damage. In addition, that professional standards, processes and methods are robust and will not result in either the loss or addition of material to an exhibit or scene at any stage (Pepper, 2005) and that exhibits are packaged in such a way to ensure that they cannot be interfered with (Cobb, 1998). The integrity of crime scenes and exhibits is central to any forensic case and is reliant on the strict adherence to policy and standards.

2.3.6 Contamination

Contamination occurs through the alteration of an exhibit or scene from its original state and thus changing its nature through the loss or addition of material, and this can be either inadvertent or deliberate (ACPO, 2006; Gallop and Stockdale, 1998). Contamination can falsely infer contact between surfaces, materials, objects, suspects and victims. The aforementioned concepts of scene security and protection in part seek to reduce contamination, and structured working at scenes and in laboratories, guards against this. Careful deployment of personnel, the use of barrier clothing and exhibit handling are essential to prevent contamination.

2.4 Records and documentation

2.4.1 The crime scene log (Book 197)

The crime scene log provides a record of information pertaining to an individual scene and its creation. For the duration of time that the scene remains open the log is used to record all people entering and leaving (Horswell, 2004) including the names of personnel, their role, the level of barrier clothing worn and specific entry and exit times (ACPO, 2006; Specialist Crime Policy Unit, 2008c). On arrival at a scene individuals working must present themselves with appropriate identification to the Police Officer holding the log. It is recommended to make a note of the times recorded by the officer to ensure consistency between personal notes and the log. Security at crime scenes is high for obvious reasons and the admittance of individuals is resultantly strict. The log is representative of the chain of evidence, integrity of the crime scene and is the starting place for the continuity of exhibits and evidence (ACPO, 2006). Once closed the log is retained by the investigative team together with the case papers (Specialist Crime Policy Unit, 2008c).

2.4.2   The Crime Scene Manager's log (Book 199)

Within the MPS, the CSM will maintain a corporate document, 'the Crime Scene Manager's Case Notes Log', which provides written evidence of forensic actions and records decisions pertaining to an incident or scene (Specialist Crime Policy Unit, 2008c). CSMs covering any aspect of an enquiry will complete their own log, but the lead CSM must hold a copy of these individual logs in order to maintain effective management over the enquiry. A copy of these notes is also passed to the MIR for inputting onto HOLMES.

This book contains records of work pertaining to crime scene management, information, observations and assessments including forensic strategies, decisions made with supporting rationales, and actions taken within the implementation of forensic strategies adopted (Specialist Crime Policy Unit, 2008c). All relevant health and safety issues and full details of risk assessments carried out are also documented here. Entries made are contemporaneous, in chronological order and are signed and dated by the CSM (Specialist Crime Policy Unit, 2008b).

2.4.3   The exhibits book (Book 170)

All exhibits seized during an investigation are recorded into books by the EO and every scene has an individual book. Exhibits are uniquely identified and allocated letters corresponding to the finder's initials and a sequential number, for example REB/1 (see Chapter 13). Exhibits have detailed descriptions including the quantity, colour, condition of the item, any endorsements and measurements. The location of where the exhibit was found is required including measurements and the name of the person who found and seized the exhibit is recorded in addition to the unique seal number of the packaging. Entries are signed and dated in accordance with the chain of evidence. The EO will maintain this log until trial, tracking each exhibit as it is moved to different forensic providers for examination and the entirety of each book is also entered onto HOLMES.

2.4.4 Notes and photos

It is the responsibility of each forensic specialist to produce their own contemporaneous notes at the scene from which they will later be required to produce a statement. The notes and details pertaining to the case should remain confidential to anyone outside the enquiry and it is expected that they are disclosed and as such must be identified and copies provided to the enquiry team. It is preferable that the only photographs taken at scenes are those by the Forensic Photographer (see Chapter 14). The CSM and the SIO will always endeavour to meet the needs of the specialist providing copies when necessary. Should specific photographs be required to accompany notes and observations then the specialist should inform the CSM, as is also the case should any photographs be taken by the specialist.

2.5 Crime scene attendance

2.5.1 Employment

Upon the request of services from the CSM, it is essential that the individual consider and divulge whether or not they are able to fully meet the requirements of the assignment. For example: Will prior engagements interrupt the time frame of the new case under consideration? Have they had any prior involvement in the case in question?

A verbal briefing is given over the phone including a description of the role that the specialist will be expected to perform, a location to meet and the contact information of individuals at the scene, commonly the CSM and EO. If appropriate, and dependent on the role for which the specialist is to be engaged, it may be necessary to discuss the resources and logistics of any equipment required. However, if the equipment required is mandatory to the role to be performed there is an expectation that the specialist will have this at their disposal. Appropriate identification must be brought to the scene to ensure access is granted.

2.5.2 Arrival

Upon arrival at the scene the specialist should approach the Police Officer holding the crime scene log who will alert the CSM or a member of the investigative team. The specialist along with their equipment will be collected and accompanied to a suitable location within the scene to receive a formal briefing. Outside the scene care should be taken when discussing the case; people commonly congregate around crime scenes therefore caution should be exercised as the presence of certain specialists may not be in the public domain.

2.5.3 Common approach path

Following the creation of a crime scene a common approach path is established; this is a route allocated for entering and exiting the scene to reduce disturbance and contamination which can result from individuals walking freely (Horswell, 2004). It is allocated taking into account areas that may hold less forensic potential or have been forensically cleared and as result may not be the most direct. It is recommended to be mindful, taking note of any guidance given by police personnel. Care should be taken not to cause unnecessary disturbance.

2.5.4 Briefing

The CSM leads the briefing and will introduce everyone present and their roles. He or she will provide further background and information on the case including the nature of the enquiry, the agreed strategy and precise details of the tasks required to be carried out. The CSM will explain the risk assessments in place and highlight any specific hazards to ensure the safety of the personnel working, and any restrictions in place. The purpose of the briefing is to ensure that everyone has a shared understanding of the case, objectives, each others' roles and risks. It provides an opportunity for questions to be addressed and clarified in addition to establishing a good working rapport among personnel. Briefings take place daily and may be revisited as and when new information or developments arise. At the end of each shift a debrief will take place to review the progress made, method, action plan and overall strategy.

2.5.5 Forensic strategy

A forensic strategy expresses the aims and objectives of the case, specific scenes and examinations; as every incident and crime scene is different, strategies are individual (ACPO, 2006). Decisions are based on the information available and specific circumstances of the case; for example, is the suspect's identity known? Forensic strategies can seek to establish if an offence has taken place, corroborate or refute individuals' accounts in addition to providing leads to an investigation such as identifying people at a scene. The strategy establishes the scope of work and examinations to be carried out and consequently determines subsequent action plans. These require regular review to assess progress and are adjusted when required to incorporate and recognise new information. It is important that specialists working at scenes have an understanding of the forensic strategy so that they are best able to determine if their methods are suitable and that the scope of the work is realistic (Bryon, 2009).

2.5.6 Protective clothing

Barrier clothing is worn to prevent contamination (Pepper, 2005), minimising contact trace transportation into the crime scene through the personnel working; and for health and safety reasons. The CSM is responsible for deciding what protective clothing is required and will instruct individuals accordingly. Basic protective clothing is disposable and designed for one use only; it consists of a face mask, two pairs of latex gloves, a scene suit with hood and overshoes. The order of putting this clothing on is important, therefore it is recommended that specialists seek advice if they are uncertain as to what to put on first and how. Talking should be avoided if not wearing a face mask and individuals should be mindful of their behaviour and actions, changing outer gloves between exhibits and any element worn if it is breeched. The basic barrier clothing is provided at the scene and the CSM will decide if it is to be retained.

2.5.7 Dynamic risk assessment

Risk assessments are conducted at all crime scenes incorporating not only personnel working there but also members of the public (ACPO, 2006). They are robust and continually reviewed, acknowledging and addressing potential hazards, risks, and where possible reducing or eliminating the danger in question completely. Commonly encountered hazards include biological and chemical substances, structural stability of buildings, uneven surfaces such as floors, slip and trip hazards, sharp items and falling debris (Anderson et al., 2008b; Pepper, 2005). The hazards presented by people are also addressed in terms of traffic, observers and outstanding suspects. Cordons, traffic control and the presence of Police Officers seek to minimise the vulnerability of personnel at scenes (Anderson et al., 2008b; Pepper, 2005). Risk assessments incorporate working safely at scenes ensuring that tools, machinery, specialist equipment, light sources and chemicals are only used by trained personnel and will not adversely affect other personnel or members of the public. The wearing of barrier clothing and additional protective equipment such as specific footwear and hard hats may be required depending on the circumstances. It is recommended that specialists recognise and bring to the attention of the CSM any risks or hazards presented by their own equipment to those around them.

2.5.8 Mortuary attendance

When attending the mortuary individuals must make representation to the Coroner's office upon arrival unless otherwise informed following which they will be directed to a room designated for the purpose of a briefing. The Pathologist, CSM and SIO will agree an order to commence the examination, formulating an examination strategy of the deceased to recover appropriate samples for further forensic examination to assist the investigation. The newest mortuaries are designed on the principle that only the Pathologist, the Anatomical Technician, CSM and Forensic Photographer are in the main post-mortem room, and other attendees are in a separate glazed viewing area equipped with communication equipment. The EO will then work in a designated area receiving exhibits through a screened hatch to package.

2.5.9   Conclusion of works

On the conclusion of work the CSM will discuss with the specialist the provision of a preliminary statement and the time frame required; further statements of work and actions surrounding exhibits will be reviewed as required. The individual will be requested to provide dates to avoid for court attendance for a set period by a witness care officer for the case, identifying holidays and pre-arranged commitments such as other trials. If required to attend court the individual will receive early warning in the months approaching the trial date and then a further overnight warning confirming the request for their evidence. Individuals wishing to refer to specifics pertaining to a case such as the photographs for teaching purposes must obtain permission from the SIO; they must also be prepared to attend case conferences to discuss findings. Invoices for services should be submitted to the EO and payment will be arranged.

2.6   Expectations

It is expected that anyone working at a crime scene does so in a professional manner taking into account their surroundings and the sensitivities of the community, and treating those around them with respect and courtesy. If a question or task is beyond an individual's expertise it is essential that they express this honestly (Menez, 2005). Wherever possible, realistic time frames for work should be given, although the authors acknowledge that this is often difficult to estimate. Crime scene work is demanding and good teamwork and rapport is crucial in order to maximise the forensic potential; the opinions, expertise and priorities of all personnel must be respected. Disputes and disagreements must be voiced professionally, resolutions sought and compromises made that are agreeable to all.

2.7   Conclusion

For the progression of multidisciplinary crime scene working and forensic investigations it is essential that specialists and police personnel increase their knowledge and understanding of each other's roles to work effectively together to meet their common goal. It is the authors' hope that both this chapter and this volume provide a firm foundation for the future, improving and streamlining forensic processes, methods and awareness.

Acknowledgements

The authors wish to thank CSM Angela Thompson and CSM Co-ordinator Joe Marchesi for their review of the manuscript, and Director of Forensic Services, Gary Pugh, OBE for his support.

References

ACPO. 2005. *Major Incident Room Standardised Administrative Procedures (MIRSAP)*. Wyboston, NCPE.

ACPO. 2006. *Murder Investigation Manual*. Wyboston, NCPE.

Anderson, A., Cox, M., Flavel, A. *et al.* 2008a. Protocols for the investigation of mass graves. In M. Cox, A. Flavel, I. Hanson *et al.* (eds) *The Scientific Investigation of Mass Graves: Towards Protocols and Standard Operating Procedures*. Cambridge University Press, Cambridge, pp. 39–105.

Anderson, A., Hanson, I., Schofield, D. *et al.* 2008a. Health and Safety. In M. Cox, A. Flavel, I. Hanson *et al.* (eds) *The Scientific Investigation of Mass Graves: Towards Protocols and Standard Operating Procedures*. Cambridge University Press, Cambridge, pp. 109–147.

Bryon, G. 2009. Forensic science support to critical and major incident investigations: A service-based approach. *The Journal of Homicide and Major Incident Investigation* 5: 75–86.

Cobb, P. 1998. Forensic Science. In P. White (ed.) *Crime Scene to Court: The Essentials of Forensic Science*. Royal Society of Chemistry, London, pp. 1–14.

Donnelly, S., Hedley, M., Loveless, T. *et al.* 2008. Scenes of crime examination. In M. Cox, A. Flavel, I. Hanson *et al.* (eds) *The Scientific Investigation of Mass Graves: Towards Protocols and Standard Operating Procedures*. Cambridge University Press, Cambridge, pp. 148–182.

Duhig, C. and Turnbull, R. 2007. Crime scene management and forensic anthropology: Observations and recommendations from the United Kingdom and international cases. In R. Ferllini (ed.) *Forensic Archaeology and Human Rights Violations*. Charles C Thomas, Springfield, IL, pp. 76–100.

Fisher, B.A.J. 1992. *Techniques of Crime Scene Investigation*, 5th edn. Elsevier Science, New York.

Gallop, A. and Stockdale, R. 1998. Trace and contact evidence. In P. White (ed.) *Crime Scene to Court: The Essentials of Forensic Science*. Royal Society of Chemistry, London, pp. 47–72.

Horswell, J. 2004. *The Practice of Crime Scene Investigation*. Taylor & Francis, London.

Hunter, J. and Cox, M. 2005. *Forensic Archaeology: Advances in Theory and Practice*. Routledge, London.

Hunter, J.R. and Knupfer, G.C. 1997. The police and judicial structure in Britain. In J. Hunter, C. Roberts and A. Martin (eds) *Studies in Crime: An Introduction to Forensic Archaeology*. Routledge, London, pp. 24–39.

Menez, L.L. 2005. The place of a forensic archaeologist at a crime scene involving a buried body. *Forensic Science International* **152**: 311–315.

Nicol, C., Innes, M., Gee, D. and Feist, A. 2004. *Reviewing murder investigations: an analysis of progress reviews from six police forces*. Home Office, London. http://library.npia.police.uk/docs/hordsolr/rdsolr2504.pdf (last accessed March 2012).

Pepper, I. 2005. *Crime Scene Investigation: Methods and Procedures*. Open University Press, Maidenhead.

Skinner, M. and Sterenberg, J. 2005. Turf wars: authority and responsibility for the investigation of mass graves. *Forensic Science International* **151**: 221–232.

Specialist Crime Policy Unit. 2008a. Specialist Crime Directorate Response and Individual Responsibilities. *London Homicide Manual*. MPS, London.

Specialist Crime Policy Unit. 2008b. Initial Response – Individual Responsibilities. *London Homicide Manual*. MPS, London.

Specialist Crime Policy Unit. 2008c. Record Keeping. *London Homicide Manual*. MPS, London.

Weston, N. 1998. The Crime Scene. In P. White (ed.) *Crime Scene to Court: The Essentials of Forensic Science*. Royal Society of Chemistry, London, pp. 15–46.

3

Forensic archaeology

Stephen Litherland,[1] Nicholas Márquez-Grant[1,2] and Julie Roberts[3]

[1] Cellmark Forensic Services, Abingdon, UK
[2] Institute of Human Sciences, School of Anthropology and Museum Ethnography, University of Oxford, Oxford, UK
[3] Cellmark Forensic Services, Chorley, UK

3.1   Introduction

This chapter is designed to introduce the role of the Forensic Archaeologist and provide guidance on the archaeological methods commonly employed at crime scenes both for the non-specialist reader and the crime scene practitioner. The perspective taken here is a UK one, deriving from the authors' own experience in police casework. A wider perspective in Europe and the United States can be found elsewhere (e.g. Hunter *et al.*, 2001; Márquez-Grant, Litherland and Roberts, 2012; Blau and Ubelaker, 2009; Dirkmaat *et al.*, 2008).

Forensic archaeology can be defined as the application of archaeological principles and methods to the search, recovery and excavation not only of human remains but also of any buried evidence within a forensic, medico-legal and/or humanitarian setting. Perhaps the most crucial point, however, is that 'the excavation of human remains results *not only* in the retrieval of the remains, but also in the reconstruction of human activity at the site and beyond' (Scott and Connor, 2001: 104; emphasis by current authors). In recent years, an increasing number of publications (e.g. Hunter and Cox, 2005; Dupras *et al.*, 2006; Connor, 2007; Blau and Ubelaker, 2009; Dirkmaat, 2012) have provided more awareness on the applications and methods employed in forensic archaeology. Similarly, the excavation of mass graves has also been a matter of publication (e.g. Haglund, Connor and Scott, 2001; Tuller and Djurić, 2006; Ferllini, 2007; Cox *et al.*, 2008).

Notoriously, one of the first recorded applications of excavation that recovered personal items and identification, coupled with anthropological examination of the human remains, took place in 1943 in the Katyn forest, where the Germans exhumed thousands of Polish victims with the aim of establishing Soviet culpability for their deaths. In the United Kingdom, it was the investigation of Stephen Jennings, whose remains were recovered from under rubble in a rural location in West Yorkshire in 1988 that set a precedent for the use of archaeological evidence in the courts (see Hunter *et al.*, 1994, for a review of these early years). Today, at least in the United Kingdom (and in many parts of the United States, usually under the umbrella of 'anthropology'), forensic archaeology is quite widely regarded as an increasingly useful discipline within criminal investigations. It has been estimated that there are usually between 50 and 70 cases where archaeology has an important role to play annually in the United Kingdom – although because of the reactive nature of this work this number is likely to be highly variable (Hunter and Cox, 2005; Cox, 2009).

There are currently probably around 20 to 30 practising forensic archaeologists in the United Kingdom who undertake casework for police forces. These practitioners are based in independent forensic providers, archaeological units, museums or universities. In addition, a small number of police forces have their own in-house archaeologist, and some Crime Scene Investigators (CSI) or Scenes of Crime Officers (SOCOs) have a degree in archaeology (see also Hunter, 2009; Márquez-Grant *et al.*, 2012).

Most of the practising forensic archaeologists in the United Kingdom are registered with the Institute for Archaeologists (IfA). Currently, accreditation, policies, guidelines and code of conduct fall under the umbrella of the IfA in which there is a special interest group for forensic archaeology. This specialist group has developed guidelines resulting also from discussions with the UK Forensic Regulator. It is the professional duty of the forensic archaeologist to comply with and fully adhere to these standards, which includes keeping abreast of advances within the subject. In the interests of providing a practical synthesis for non-specialists and the development of a single practice-based terminology, these IfA standards (Powers and Sibun, 2011) are quoted extensively in the sections below.

The request for a forensic archaeologist to become involved in an enquiry may come from a number of sources within a police force such as, for example, a Senior CSI or Forensic Investigator or SOCO – these titles are largely interchangeable between different police forces in the United Kingdom at present – a SSM (Scientific Support Manager), a Forensic Coordinator, or the OIC (Officer in Charge) (see also Márquez-Grant *et al.*, 2012; Hunter and Cox, 2005; Hunter, 2009). A police force may also contact regional NPIA (National Policing Improvement Agency) advisors who can consult a database of registered Expert Advisors from a wide range of professions, including archaeology. In any case, the archaeologist is ultimately responsible to the SIO (Senior Investigating Officer) who has absolute responsibility for any investigation. As will be seen later, the types of request are varied, but usually fall within the remit of the search, location and recovery of buried bodies or items.

At a potential scene of crime, the forensic archaeologist may often work within a large team of police, civilian and specialist staff (see Chapter 2). During a search it is common to work under the direction of specialist search staff (PolSA), but also liaising with CSIs (and detectives). If the search is successful and thereby turns into a crime scene then commonly the scientific support (CSIs) will take over the management of the work and will then usually control the process of production of exhibits of items found and ensure that full photographic and chain of custody records are maintained. A photographer (see Chapter 14) and exhibits officer (see Chapter 13) should be regarded as the absolute minimum in terms of support staff at a small scene. It is also best practice for two archaeologists (or alternatively an anthropologist with archaeological experience when dealing with the excavation of human remains) to provide mutual support and assistance at a scene. The archaeologist will provide advice to the police team and the reasons for any decisions made should be fully documented by the archaeologist.

3.2   Forensic archaeology at a crime scene

At a potential crime scene, the forensic archaeologist may be required to advise on the:

- search, location, excavation and recording of clandestine graves;
- search for other buried items including firearms and drugs;
- investigation of a suspicious area of sunken and disturbed ground as reported by a member of the public;
- exhumation for cold case reviews;
- contextual dating of bones.

He or she may also get involved in recording surface scatter scenes of human remains, assist in fire scene reconstruction in conjunction with other specialists, or be involved in mass fatality incidents (e.g. see Dirkmaat, 2012).

The archaeologist brings a broad set of skills to a potential crime scene and is there to assist this process in the most effective and efficient way possible in accordance with the Police and Criminal Evidence Act 1984. The involvement of the forensic archaeologist should also ensure that a body or item can be searched for and recovered faster and in such a manner that it both maximises and preserves the available evidence for later presentation in court. The forensic archaeologist therefore should be equipped through training and experience with a particular and unique set of skills including knowledge of surveying techniques, search methods, field-craft and landscape analysis, processes of site formation, recording and excavation techniques, use of heavy equipment, artefact collection, sampling for other evidence types such as soils or pollen, basic awareness of human and non-human anatomy, and an ability to collect, preserve and recover human remains in whatever form these may be presented – but most importantly he or she should be able to creatively apply these skills in a flexible way to a particular forensic context (e.g. Hunter *et al.*, 1994; Owsley, 2001; Dupras *et al.*, 2006; Cheetham and Hanson, 2009; see also Márquez-Grant, Acinas Robledo and Sánchez-Sánchez, 2011; Márquez-Grant *et al.*, 2012). They must also be aware of the validity and usefulness of the evidence as well as police procedures at the crime scene (see Chapter 2), including the production of exhibits (see Chapter 13), understanding the importance of continuity and maintaining the integrity of the evidence, and working within a medico-legal framework. These skills cannot be learnt in the classroom, but instead are acquired through years of practical experience. For example, when directing and supervising the stripping of the topsoil of a garden in a search, the archaeologist will monitor these excavations for any disturbance or features[1] that may translate into a potential target by their ability to discern delicately portrayed features in soils of many colours and textures. Importantly, in the context of a negative search where nothing suspicious is found they can also dictate the level at which stripping can be safely stopped and investigation at the site be confidently concluded.

In many scenarios and for various reasons archaeologists may also find themselves an 'acting point' in terms of being at the scene to recover the other ecological evidence types referred to in this volume (e.g. Chapters 10, 11 and 12). Here it is important to recognise the limits of your professional knowledge and obtain appropriate specialist advice as to the best methods of recovery and recording required, if it is not practical for another specialist to be present at the scene within the time frame available.

As stated by Cheetham and Hanson (2009: 146), 'stratigraphic excavation is the cornerstone of the recovery of evidential data from forensic excavation'. They inform that stratigraphy[2] is the evidence that can provide an insight into the sequence of events leading to disposal and burial. It will also provide dating of evidence where possible. Archaeology is a destructive process and not excavating and recording stratigraphy reliably has negative effects with regard to the reliability of evidence. For example, if a grave (the grave cut and its fill) is not archaeologically excavated to exactly the point that a perpetrator originally dug it and is either overcut or undercut, there is both a potential for the loss of crucial evidence (e.g. tool marks) or evidential contamination so that any evidence recovered cannot be confidently linked to the sequence of events associated with the making of the grave.

---

[1] A 'feature' is defined as a physical event that can be seen in the ground; this may be a negative event such as the cutting of a grave, or a positive feature which has been built such as a garden wall.

[2] The word 'stratigraphy' has been taken from geological science in archaeology to refer to man-made contexts as well as natural soils. It is used to find the order of development of a site which enables at least relative dating to be achieved.

Importantly, the forensic archaeologist should also be able to advise on the dating of a particular activity such as the excavation of a grave and the deposition of a body, and at the very least be able to provide a broad chronology in conjunction with other evidence types, which is based upon the stratigraphic sequence. This a complicated subject for the non-specialist reader and the following definitions should be taken with many caveats, but put in simple terms excavation should provide a *terminus ante-quem* (a time after which an activity cannot have taken place or, in other words, the latest date something can be) and a *terminus post-quem* (a time before which an activity cannot have taken place or, in other words, providing a minimum date) for the deposition of a body. For example, if it can be demonstrated that a coin in the pocket of a buried victim is dated to 2011 then that person cannot have been buried before the date of the coin, but would have been buried either the same year (2011) or after *(terminus post-quem)*. This knowledge can enable an archaeologist to confidently eliminate a search area quickly without having to dig down to a layer created in geological time such as glacially deposited gravels. For instance, in a recent case there was a search for the body of a person who had been missing for just under 20 years; by using background research – looking at old maps and the surrounding buildings in the search area – it was established that the search area had once been a nineteenth-century farmyard, therefore by stripping down to the original level of the farmyard that search could confidently and quickly be established as being negative (i.e. absence of a body) as undisturbed nineteenth-century layers could not contain a 20-year-old burial.

By its very nature a grave is a very good example of Locard's Exchange Principle between perpetrator and victim ('every contact leaves a trace'). Excavation of a grave using archaeological techniques by an experienced forensic archaeologist can elucidate many circumstances surrounding a burial. For example, the archaeologist can observe:

- How was the grave dug and with what?
- How was it backfilled? Are there materials and fills that are foreign to that particular location?
- Did the perpetrator leave any traces in or around the grave such as footwear or tool marks?
- Has there been any subsequent disturbance?
- Was the grave left open for some time before, during or after the body was placed in it?

In a recent case where a body was buried over 1 m deep in the back garden of a house, the size and shape of the grave dug explained the angle and position of the body, and provided an indication of the minimum number of individuals probably required to dig the grave and what tools they would probably have used. From reading its shape and profile it was possible to see that there were different phases in the construction of the grave, which was opened first, then enlarged and a step added within the cut to excavate deeper still (thereby creating a stepped grave), all of which was dug through underlying mudstone geology which is very difficult to excavate.

Finally, there are a number of situations and pre-requisites associated with forensic archaeological casework that the archaeologist should feel comfortable to undertake. These include situations where there are fleshed, decomposed and often badly smelling remains. It also includes the requirement to produce witness statements and act as an expert witness, and the ability to work within budgetary and time constraints.

The several stages in the progress of an archaeological search or excavation from crime scene to court are outlined below.

3.3   Pre-scene attendance

3.3.1   Initial contact

This first stage in the life of an investigation is crucial in beginning to outline the likely circumstances and nature of all subsequent work. This initial contact should be well documented. This includes documenting who is contacting the archaeologist, time and date; the nature of the case; location of briefing or scene and agreed time to attend; any logistical issues and equipment; and the potential of archaeological input amongst other information (after Powers and Sibun, 2011).

At this stage, probable equipment and logistical requirements can be outlined so that these can be in place when work at a scene begins. In addition, the likely personnel requirements can also be discussed and the start of a strategy to integrate all the various specialist requirements be compiled.

It is also the duty of the forensic archaeologist to ensure that they can be available at the shortest and most opportune time in order for work to begin. For this to happen the archaeologist should ideally have all the necessary equipment and paperwork to carry out a basic excavation readily to hand, since often the initial request for work to be carried out is urgent, as the custodial clock for holding a suspect for instance may already have begun to tick.

The equipment would generally include as a minimum: a spade, a shovel, a digging mattock, a hand shovel, buckets, sieves (10 mm and 5 mm), 3-inch pointing trowels, plasterer's leaf trowel, disposable teaspoons and spatulae, paintbrushes, assorted sizes of plastic and paper tamper evident bags and pots, tarpaulin, 6-inch nails, survey arrows, North arrow, builder's line, a line level and plumb bob, hand tapes, 30 m or 50 m survey tapes, Bulldog clips, pencils (6H), pens, erasers, weatherproof permatrace paper, drawing board, masking tape, field recording sheets (e.g. context sheets, body recovery sheets; see Appendix), camera and photographic scales, compass. In addition, personal protective equipment (PPE) must be worn as and when required and appropriate (e.g. safety helmet, work boots).

3.3.2 Briefing

After the initial call or request to attend a scene, there should be a briefing usually undertaken with all interested parties being present. This will commonly take place at a police station close to the scene, or alternatively actually at the potential scene. As Powers and Sibun (2011) indicate, at a briefing the archaeologist should discuss:

- the potential for archaeological input or scope;

- any health and safety concerns;

- an archaeological strategy for the search and/or excavation, to be discussed with the CSM and considering other specialists who may be present;

- issues relating to PPE and any support services (e.g. photography) or equipment required.

This is often the situation in which the archaeologist is provided with details concerning a case, including previous actions, witness information and other information as deemed to be required by the SIO. It is important to establish the method of teamwork and the hierarchy and responsibilities of all concerned. Health and safety strategies, which must be flexible and dynamic, will also be outlined. The archaeologist should also advise as to any legal protection or heritage issues possibly relating to a scene.

3.4 Scene attendance

3.4.1 Search

In a search situation it is important to be fully aware of all specialist input and advise as to the applicability of using the various evidence types outlined in this volume, and others as directed by specialist search officers (PolSA) who will usually be coordinating all such work.

Prior to or during a search, for instance of a clandestine grave, the forensic archaeologist must undertake a desk-based assessment (DBA) or evaluation of an area by obtaining background information on the area including any known archaeological features in order to understand or even define the parameters to be searched. For this, it will be necessary to produce an archaeological search strategy in consultation with the PolSA team or CSM and taking into consideration other specialists (see Powers and Sibun, 2011). A DBA may also be undertaken after the excavation and scene attendance as this may help to understand drift geology of the area.

Various forms of background research can help to understand the development of a search area which can input into overall search strategy. Some of the specialist skills that the archaeologist can bring to a search are provided below.

3.4.1.1   Aerial photography, satellite and thermal imagery

Through background and training, archaeologists are familiar with both the uses and limitations of aerial photography, including where to track down various more obscure sources of historic aerial photography. In addition, there are various specialist providers who deal with this important source of information.

Changes caused by disturbances of the ground such as burials can persist for thousands of years and in the right conditions are visible on aerial images, a technique which has been used by archaeologists for over a century (Barber, 2011). Recent aerial photographs and satellite imagery can also be compared to older images to assess what changes there have been in the landscape.

Aerial imagery can be used to survey relatively large areas of land where a field search may be impractical. Satellite, helicopter, aeroplane or drone-based mounting platforms are available to police forces, and specialist interpretative advice and hardware is available in the United Kingdom through JARIC (the Joint Air Reconnaissance Intelligence Centre). Specialist equipment such as thermal imagery can also detect the heat given off by a decomposing body in certain conditions and within certain time frames, and may be useful in the location of more recent burials or decomposing surface remains (Servello, 2010). Air-mounted forms of radar-based ground survey (LIDAR) can also provide a very accurate, detailed and rapid survey of large areas of landscapes and, importantly, are also capable of reading the ground through tree cover. This information when used in combination with specialist mapping facilities is a great aid in the planning and definition of specific search areas.

There are various readily available sources of aerial imagery information that are downloadable from the Internet which can also be of use in planning the search of an area such as the back garden of a house. However, a major limitation of these sources is that they are not precisely dated, and may commonly have been taken over any point in the last five years or so. An often overlooked source of aerial imagery is that taken for planning purposes by local authorities. Although coverage is variable across the country, it is common for this type of survey to be undertaken in the United Kingdom roughly every three to five years and so it can be useful for older cases. The resolution of this digital imagery (widely and increasingly utilised within the last 10 years or so) is constantly improving and it is properly dated, though older conventional imagery can also be of use. For example, in a recent case there was information that a neonate had been buried in a graveyard several years ago. Examination of a series of conventional aerial photographs (in this case held by the National Monuments Record) established that ground conditions there had changed considerably over the time frame in question and most particularly when compared with the present landscape, and therefore the search parameters were able to be enhanced to reflect these changes. In another recent example, a body was discovered on an embankment close to a junction of a motorway. The local planning department was able to provide a dated series of aerial images which went someway towards explaining why this particular site was chosen (e.g. access routes, concealment through vegetation, etc.). In another case, the circumstances of some unidentified surface scattered human remains found within a disused industrial plant were explicable in terms of dating when a very secure boundary fence to the property had been built.

3.4.1.2 Maps and computer search engines

Maps exist in many forms and with several different functions. Reference is made to geology and soils maps in Chapter 12, and these are also of use to archaeologists in considering potential deposition sites. For example, if a search area includes soils or geology that are difficult or impossible to excavate by hand, these areas can then be downgraded as probable areas of clandestine burial. Land-use maps can also help to define the level of occupancy of a landscape. Conventional mapping (usually undertaken in the United Kingdom by the Ordnance Survey (OS)) can be of use to the archaeologist in a number of ways to help frame a search by providing focus through the probable elimination or downgrading of some areas of suspicion such as service trenches, archaeological and natural features; or conversely to produce a series of targets for deposition. For instance, examination of older mapping may help to locate mine shafts or entrances in a relict industrial landscape, or show the location of other buried features such as ice houses.

Mapping at 1:10000 or 6 inches to the mile is often of most use in a large-scale search coordination as the level of detail is good, including contours, building size and the boundaries of fields. Often the most detailed historic mapping available is the 1:2500 or 25 inch series which covers the whole of the United Kingdom usually dating from around the 1880s onwards in a series of roughly decadal editions (although for urban areas this can be as good as 1:500). These can be of help in a number of different ways such as when used in conjunction with aerial photography to reconstruct the development of landscape such as a back garden to show when various structures were built or account for difference in land use.

Archaeological online search engines are also available in the United Kingdom such as the national archaeological database (e.g. Archaeology Data Service or ADS) which lists ancient sites and monuments, including burial grounds, and also records previous archaeological work undertaken in a given area. Likewise, soils, land use and historic map search engines are available (e.g. www.old-maps.co.uk; www.landis.org.uk/soilscapes) which can be of help in making a rapid assessment of a site, which can be useful at the briefing stage. For instance an individual was believed to have been buried in an area immediately adjacent to a historic church burial ground. It was possible to establish from looking at a series of historic maps that this area was never part of the graveyard and so the possibility of locating other historic graves there could be confidently eliminated.

3.4.1.3 Geophysical survey

Geophysical survey in forensics (e.g. see Killam, 2004; Dupras et al., 2006) can be used to indicate areas of disturbance beneath the ground, which are not visible on the ground surface. These 'targets' then have to be investigated by excavation in order to confirm whether or not they are graves. The use of geophysical survey is a specialist subject in its own right and is discussed in Chapter 12, but some general information can be given here as a guide, as archaeologists commonly work with this type of specialist provider. In general, three main types of geophysical survey are used in archaeology: resistivity, magnetic survey and ground penetrating radar:

- **Resistivity** measures resistance to an electrical current passed between sets of electrodes placed into the ground. It is possible to conduct a survey of an average back garden in a day or so. It works well over graves of long-standing duration but does not tend to work accurately if a target is several metres deep, or in very dry or very wet environments.

- **Magnetic survey** commonly measures anomalies in the earth's magnetic field that may be caused by the mixing of top and subsoil, silting up of the grave, ferrous metal, or burning; but it does not work well where there is a lot of background 'noise' at the scene from overhead power cables, or ferrous metal such as fences or on the operator.

- **Ground penetrating radar (GPR)** emits radio-waves into the ground which are bounced back from subsurface features. Depending on the type of instrument used it can penetrate to greater depths than the other two methods and give a detailed 3D profile. Most importantly it can see through and detect voids in walls and floors, and is less affected by background 'noise'. It works well over sand, gravel, limestone, granite and ice, but it does not work well in clay soils.

3.4.1.4   Field craft

The archaeologist has commonly been trained in reading a landscape in order to interpret historic changes. This can be of use in prioritising potential search targets or eliminating or downgrading others that are probably historic. Burying human remains in the ground will alter the profile of the soil and create a dynamic micro-environment. Disturbances may cause the ground to become wetter, or more loosely compacted and free draining. It will also set in motion changes in the overlying vegetation. Specific changes to the topography and vegetation are as follows:

- Topography
  - look for areas which appear to be out of place, such as humps and bumps and hollows which do not fit in with the natural landscape;
  - as the body decomposes the ground will sink and defined edges may be seen;
  - the soil overlying a grave may be cracked;

- deposits of spoil[3] may be present around the grave;

- these changes may persist for many months depending on the environment.

- Vegetation

  - in a burial the organic content of the soil may increase. Initially this will tend to be toxic to the overlying vegetation and it will look brown, stunted and unhealthy;

  - as the body decomposes, however, nutrients are produced at beneficial levels. This will cause plants to grow better and appear more lush, green and taller than those surrounding them;

  - different plants that prefer organic rich soil or disturbed ground, such as nettles, may take over.

All of these changes are dependent on the time of year, type of environment (e.g. desert, woodland), depth of burial and any coverings around the body or burial.

Where targets have been identified in a search (Figure 3.1) these are prioritised in consultation with the specialist search advisors (PolSA). Other police resources might also have been used (e.g. cadaver dogs) and these and the archaeological resources can be combined to show the targets with most potential. It will then be necessary to test these targets, working from the most likely to the least likely for a clandestine grave. This is commonly done using many of the excavation techniques outlined in the following Section 3.4.2 on recovery, but is often limited to half-sectioning of a target only, or even the cutting of a slot though the centre of a target to try to ascertain the presence of a body or not, its likely cause, and either eliminate it as a potential burial or continue to excavate to define it in more detail.

Finally, search may be undertaken in a number of systematic ways, including dividing the search area into transects, grids or zones, for example.

3.4.2 Recovery

If the search is successful and a target is positive or, alternatively, if good intelligence information leads to the identification of a probable area, then the forensic archaeologist must (after Powers and Sibun, 2011):

- record his or her actions at the scene, including individuals present, strategy, when entered and departed the scene, etc.;

---

[3] 'Spoil' can be defined as the excess soil and other intrusive material such as bricks or stones that is created through the digging of a hole in the ground.

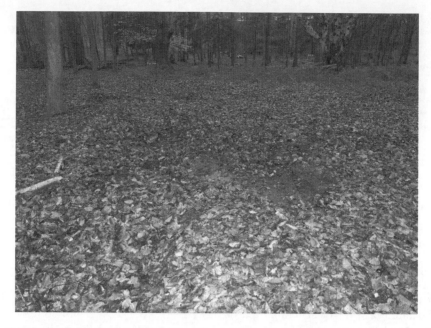

Figure 3.1 Potential target in the search of three clandestine graves in a training exercise. In this image, disturbed autumn surface vegetation layers and spoil. There is also sinking of the ground and a number of tree stumps which potentially could serve as grave markers. (To see a colour version of this figure, please see Plate 3.1.)

- ensure that the feature is investigated using the most appropriate archaeological technique for that specific case (e.g. hand excavated with a trowel; machine excavated);

- maintain stratigraphic integrity, aim to maximize the recovery of evidence and undertake appropriate recording (written notes, illustrations such as plans, section drawings and sketches, and photographs);

- advise on samples to be collected and advise on the retention of the excavated soil (e.g. in bins and clearly labelled with context number);

- understand scene protocols, the entry and exit routes (common approach path) and discuss any strategy or actions with the CSM, including protocols to avoid contamination (e.g. Tyvek suit, hairnets, facemasks, gloves), the taking of photographs (see Chapter 14) and production of exhibits (see Chapter 13).

3.4.2.1   *Buried remains*

Prior to excavating a potential feature with buried human remains, and depending on experience, an archaeologist may want to excavate a test pit to understand the geology of the area (e.g. what is natural or what is not natural) and this can be done if possible, for example 5 m away from the potential target. Undertaking this test pit, however, will depend on the situation, the case and logistics as well as experience. In any case, a prior knowledge of the geology of the area is be recommended. When proceeding to excavate the actual target the forensic archaeologist, in the case of a clandestine grave, should (in approximate sequence from beginning to end):

1. locate the grave within the scene using GPS, tapes or a total station (see 'Recording' below);

2. take environmental samples from the soil overlying and around the potential grave;

3. use the flat edge of the trowel to scrape back the surface soil to expose the grave cut in plan;

4. draw a scaled plan and photograph;

5. excavate only within the grave cut (i.e. excavate the fill) in order to reveal the original base and sides of the grave;

6. remove one half of the grave first down to the level that human remains can confidently be identified, working systematically from one end of the grave and progressing towards the other for each layer. This is called 'half-sectioning'. The half-section through the grave allows a picture of the nature of its formation to be obtained and may show evidence of its having been dug and left open for a time frame. Whether different materials have been imported into the backfill of the grave or whether it has subsequently been re-dug is all interpretable from observation of different layers and the sequence of deposits within a grave. If the grave is deep or complex, it may be necessary to excavate in arbitrary spits (commonly between 10 and 20 cm in depth and each assigned a number);

7. pay attention to layers and any colour changes in soil. These may represent separate burial events, secondary digging and backfilling, or soil brought in from elsewhere on the spade or footwear of the perpetrator;

8. undertake a section drawing (remember you will require builder's string, a line level, measuring tapes and drawing equipment);

9. record the position of evidence according to layer. This may involve assigning context numbers to the layers.[4] The soil around the body must be given a different context number and kept separately. This latter is recommended mainly for two reasons: (a) it is a biohazard and this should be clearly labelled; and (b) it may contain trace evidence and human tissue (e.g. nails, hair, etc.);

---

[4] A 'context' (or 'stratigraphic unit' as most commonly known in other countries) is the overarching archaeological word for a unique event, it may be a man-made layer, geological deposit or a feature such as a grave cut or a garden wall.

10. sieve and retain all grave fill, look for teeth, hairs, cartilage, small bones such as the hyoid or carpal bones or epiphyses (in the case of young or immature skeletons); excavate the other half of the grave;

11. examine the base and the sides of the grave – there may be evidence of tool marks or footprints that can be cast – take soil and pollen samples from the base and the sides of the grave and from each layer dug;

12. before lifting the remains record:

    – depth of burial;

    – orientation of body;

    – whether the body is lying on its front (prone), on its back (supine) or side;

    – position of arms, legs and head;

    – relationship to other evidence;

    – any coverings;

    – what lies above and below the burial including soil, stones, vegetation, adipocere or other body fluids that might indicate decomposition *in situ*;

    – missing or damaged body parts or individual bones.

After the above, the remains will be removed and further excavation continued until the base of the grave is defined (see below). This will also require soil sampling and proper documentation (e.g. plan drawing) (Figures 3.2 and 3.3).

3.4.2.2   *Removing the human remains from the grave*

How this is achieved is highly dependent on the state of preservation of the remains and the burial environment. If the body is still articulated (i.e. held together by soft tissue), the following is advisable, although it depends on the logistics at the scene and nature of the deposition:

- roll up a body sheet. Roll the body onto its side in the grave, tuck the sheet under the body as far as it will go, then roll the body back onto the sheet and pull the sheet through to the other side;

- lift the body out on the sheet and place it in the body bag;

- collect any residue from beneath the body, place in separate container, label and keep with body bag;

- sieve the soil beneath and around the body, paying particular attention to the regions of the hands, feet, neck and head;

- if the hands, head and feet appear 'unstable' tie bags over them prior to rolling the body onto the sheet.

(a): Prior to excavation

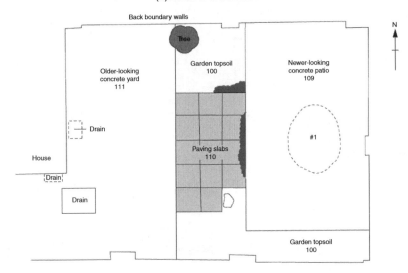

(b): At the end of the search showing positions of the grave, roll of underlay and roll of carpet

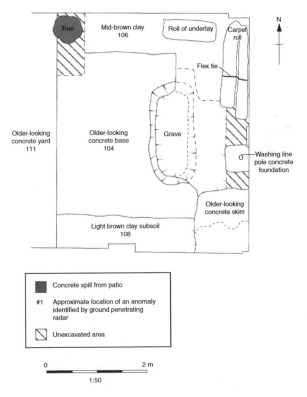

Figure 3.2 Pre-excavation plan and excavation plan in the case of a clandestine grave in a back garden.

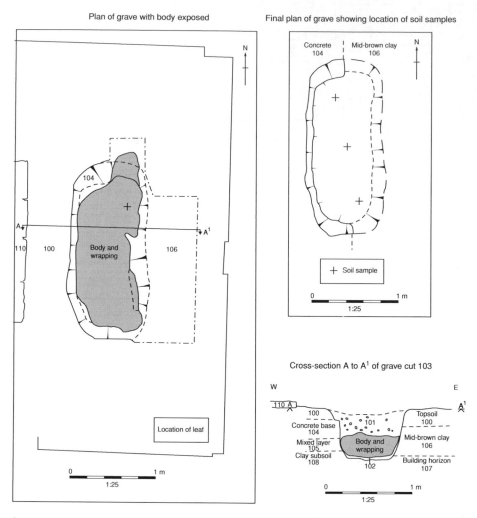

Figure 3.3 Plan and section drawing of the grave, as well as the location of soil samples taken at the base of the grave.

If the body is skeletonised:

- ensure that all the bones are fully exposed before trying to remove them. Do not pull bones out of the ground;

- lift bones individually;

- lightly brush off loose soil and retain;

- bag right and left bones separately and clearly label, this is particularly important if remains are juvenile;

- bag the right fourth rib separately;

- sieve all soil as above;

- pierce bags to reduce condensation;

- place in boxes and surround with bubble wrap.

For transportation, it is advisable that the skull (cranium and mandible) are contained in a box but within the body bag or packed in the body bag supported by acid-free tissue (e.g. paper roll). Due to the importance of the hip bones for sex and age-at-death estimation (see Chapter 4), these may also be packaged securely within the body bag. Good packaging will protect the bones from possible fracturing during transportation from the scene to the mortuary.

If remains are very fragmented and/or burnt:

- record as much data as possible in the ground (if at all possible in conjunction with an anthropologist at the scene, see Chapter 4);

- lift in a block and place in a suitable receptacle (the type of container will depend upon whether the context is wet or dry);

- collect soil above, below and surrounding deposit and send to the appropriate specialist, with the bulk sample, for processing.

Depending on the nature of the context, the area to be excavated containing burnt remains may be excavated according to zones or grids. This will allow for a better understanding of the location of the remains and contribute to understanding body position and orientation.

3.4.3   Recording remains

Accurate recording of the position of bodies, body parts, ballistics and associated evidence at the scene can:

- assist in reconstruction of events surrounding death;

- assist in reconstruction of events surrounding burial or post-depositional activity;

- assist with assignation of body parts to correct body in mass fatality incidents and/or where remains are scattered.

The following principles apply whether the remains are buried, or scattered on the ground surface:

- photograph (or even video-record) the scene, the grave, and the remains, pre- and post-excavation;

- recording may be done digitally using a total station, or manually using tape measures;

- whichever method is used, first set up a datum point – a point of reference from which all measurements will be taken;

- horizontally – if you are using tapes, you can either create a physical grid of quadrants within which you will record the position of the evidence, or measure 'off-sets' at right angles from a base line running between two points that are related to established features, such as the corner of a field or a building;

- vertically – establish a horizontal datum line across the grave above the unexcavated half-section face and measure all details and the profile of the cut measuring at right angles to this line from known points (you will also need to record the position of the line horizontally). Depths can be measured using a tape measure;

- alternatively, the whole scene and details of the grave and the evidence can be measured quickly and accurately using a survey instrument such as a total station or laser scanner, the total station has functions to measure height, distance and angles, and can produce a 3D map of the area.

3.5   Case studies

In this section we present a selection of case studies that serve to illustrate the range of potential work (after Márquez-Grant *et al.*, 2011, 2012; see also case studies in Hunter and Cox, 2005). As can be seen, although the main role of the forensic archaeologist is the search, detection or location and recovery of human remains, as a grave is a locus of contact between victim and perpetrator/s, he or she is often also concerned with many of the other evidence types discussed in this volume.

- *Search for the presumed body of a named individual who has been missing for some time and where there is very little intelligence information about the whereabouts of the body.* On occasions there is no specific information regarding the disappearance of an individual. This is probably one of the most common requests by police forces and on a lot of occasions the results are negative. For example in the case of an individual missing for 10 years, after a series of police investigations a warrant was obtained to check the house where he was living at the time of his disappearance. This included an examination of a back garden and patio, where ground penetrating radar had identified several targets or anomalies. A visual inspection of the area was made, looking for changes in the topography, areas of soil disturbance, spoil or broken roots. The most likely targets from both methods of search were then targeted by means of excavation. These anomalies proved negative for human remains but to be certain of this the topsoil across the entire garden was then stripped away by a mechanical machine (a mini-digger). One case with positive results followed concerns raised by a neighbourhood in relation to a neighbour they had not seen for several months. A visual search of the back garden identified two likely features and exploration of the most likely area revealed a body buried under several layers of concrete.

- *To investigate an area where there is good intelligence information regarding allegations that a body has been buried in a particular place.* In one such case there was good evidence that there were human remains in the back garden and patio of a property (Figures 3.2. and 3.3). GPR identified a potential target under an area of concrete. After the removal of concrete the area was trowelled back and an oval feature was identified. This was excavated to reveal a clothed skeletonised human body wrapped in fabric. After the removal of the remains the grave was completely excavated and soil samples were taken from the base of the grave. The entire back garden was then excavated with the aim of investigating any other evidence relating to the identification of the deceased, a murder weapon or any other information that might be thought as relevant.

- *Search for potential clandestine burial in a large area (e.g. forest, field).* On occasions, the search of a missing person has to cover large areas. In one such case, pollen and soil evidence from the suspect's car allowed the search area to be narrowed down and after a visual inspection of a wood noting topography, vegetation and soil changes the archaeologist was able to prioritise an area of suspicion. Here the earth had 'sunk' and there was evidence of loose soil and vegetation. On excavation this turned out to be a grave over 1.5m deep in which lay the body of the missing person. In this case it was necessary to remove one side of the grave after recording in order to allow easier access for the removal of the body.

- *Accidental discovery of unburied human remains.* On occasions partially exposed bodies are accidentally discovered and the archaeologist will assist an anthropologist at the scene to record the context of the remains. In one particular example skeletonised buried remains were uncovered by construction workers reinforcing the footings of a building. The forensic archaeologist was able to establish that the remains were in fact a burial that was cut by the foundations of the nineteenth-century extension and were therefore not of concern. In another example, a body was found amongst a rubbish tip in an urban area. The archaeologist called to attend the scene was able to identify the context and dating of the deposition in relation to the surrounding rubbish.

Listed above are probably the most common types of requests that police forces make to forensic archaeologists. However, there are also a number of other requests that we have worked on in recent years including exhumation. Here police may need to exhume a body either for a cold case review or in the light of new evidence concerning the death of an individual or in order to obtain a sample for DNA. The archaeologist can advise on the safe and practical ways of achieving efficient recovery, particularly in a graveyard where there may be closely spaced burials or where the human remains have been disturbed by collapsed coffin or root action amongst other factors. They can also advise on soil conditions and potential requirement for such things as a mechanical pump to drain out water and potential for remains to have shifted within the grave. The archaeologist with some knowledge of taphonomy – the analysis of the process of decomposition – will also be able to comment on likely state of preservation of remains and therefore advise on requirements in the mortuary. One example was a cold case review where the victim had died 19 years previously and had been kept in a freezer at the mortuary for three years, and so had been buried for 16 years; but since crucial parts of the body were missing, in this case the head and both hands, identification was unsuccessful at the time of his death. The body was exhumed to see if further analysis could be undertaken including DNA and stable isotope analysis.

3.6   Reporting and court testimony

As established in the UK guidelines by the Specialist Forensic Archaeology Interest Group (Powers and Sibun, 2011) from the Institute for Archaeologists, the forensic archaeologist must produce a formal report of his or her findings. This report should contain information on background to the case, the actions and decisions taken at the scene, information on the excavation strategy and methods used, the results of the excavation and interpretation of the findings, and any additional information required to comply with disclosure obligations. In England and Wales, the specialist should comply with the Crown Prosecution Service (CPS) guidance on expert witnesses' obligations on disclosure (Annex K of The Disclosure Manual, 2005: http://www.cps.gov.uk/legal/d_to_g/disclosure_manual/). Finally, the archaeologist must ensure that the requirements outlined in the Criminal Procedure Rules (2010, Part 33) are met (in Powers and Sibun, 2011).

All records related to the excavation need to be stored in a secured location and are available to the defence if a case comes to court. The report should be both logical and clear to the lay person with no archaeological knowledge and should include:

- Police reference number or Operation name, archaeology case number.

- Qualifications of the expert as well as experience and membership of any relevant associations. This is to prove credibility of the witness.

- Non-technical summary. A brief summary outlining the results is very useful for the non-specialist reader.

- Introduction. The introduction may indicate background information, request for archaeological input (e.g. to attend a scene), nature of the job, dates on which scene attended and times, use of assistants, etc.

- Background. Usually background to the case and a description of the location to be searched. Grid reference, geology and past land use is also worth including.

- Methods/Technical Notes. Methods employed (e.g. hand excavation with trowel), recording protocols, definitions (e.g. 'stratigraphy'), whether it was excavated in wet or dry conditions, search according to zones or grids, etc.

- Results of scene attendance. Results should include observations made throughout the excavation process, strategies and decisions undertaken, any features identified and excavated and their interpretation, etc. Remember that describing what is absent is also as important as what is present; absence of a body or negative results must be stated too.

- Supplementary analysis including dating from artefacts is also essential where appropriate.

- Discussion and conclusions. Conclusions may be relating to the discovery of the remains but also on the dating of the grave/feature. It may also be on specific artefacts found that may lead to showing the involvement of a third party. It may be necessary at times, to be prepared to consider new information (e.g. dating of artefacts recovered within a fill) and produce supplementary reports if required. The strength of evidence may also be presented in a number of ways (e.g. Bayesian approach).

- Bibliography (if applicable).

- Appendix. Here, for example, the expert can include notes on quantification of records and samples retained, exhibits created at the scene should also be listed, plans, section drawings and photographs may also be included.

It is also vitally important that the report is peer reviewed or checked by another forensic archaeologist of similar standing.

3.6.1 Court appearance

On occasions, archaeologists may be required to attend court. In fact, all field notes, sketches, drawings and plans, and any recording forms will be court-admissible and made available to the defence. This may be as a request from the prosecution to summarise some of the findings and to emphasize certain discoveries, results or interpretations; or it might be by the defence when there might be dispute about something included in the statement. Cross-examination may relate particularly to the dating of a feature, to how the feature was dug and its dimensions, on the material that was used to backfill the grave, the tasks undertaken, qualifications and experience, and techniques employed. The archaeologist must be competent and confident to appear in court and be unbiased and impartial to either the prosecution or defence. It is expected that their appearance and behaviour will be most appropriate, that questions will be answered truthfully (remember the expert witness will have oathed or affirmed to tell the truth), the evidence delivered in a comprehensive manner, and that the expert will stick to their remit for that particular case and above all within her or his field of expertise. Questions within the remit of the archaeologist may include the way in which the body was deposited, whether the grave required considerable amount of time–effort to construct, whether it was deep or shallow, whether any tool marks could point to possible tools used to dig the grave. The archaeologist may also be asked to comment on any evidence seized by him or her (see also Powers and Sibun, 2011; Márquez-Grant *et al.*, 2012; Dilley, 2005).

Finally, the defence barristers can also appoint an archaeologist to produce a report on the case presented by the prosecution.

3.7 Conclusion

To sum up the points above, the archaeologist is there to advise on the search and where human remains have been located; he or she is there to assist the police in the recovery of the remains, sometimes alongside the anthropologist (this depends on whether the remains are fully fleshed, or whether they are semi-skeletonised or decomposed). He or she should maximise the recovery of other evidence, including other ecology-type evidence. The appropriate and correct recording should be undertaken since archaeology is a destructive process and the records may be used in court by the prosecution and defence. Overall, it is the recording and understanding of the context in which the remains were found that will provide a more accurate interpretation of the events surrounding burial and deposition. Dating is also another important aspect to which the archaeologist can contribute. These skills and expertise are increasingly being acknowledged, and training, lectures and seminars given by archaeologists to police officers throughout the country, as well as the attendance of police staff at archaeological conferences, has been a great stimulus for awareness. Certainly, with an increasing published literature, the important role of archaeologists in human rights investigations and their contribution from crime scene to court is further evidence in recent years that forensic archaeology can provide an invaluable and much needed input.

The importance of forensic archaeology is certainly growing, not only with regard to the number of courses at universities, practitioners and involvement in casework, but certainly too with regard to training and research. Research in forensic archaeology is encouraged, for example the authors' work in progress is examining the time and effort placed into excavating a grave, testing grave excavation in different soil environments and by people of different physique, age and sex, and even-handedness.

It is hoped that this paper can serve not only as a further contribution to the already published literature on the importance of forensic archaeology, its applications and its value in crime scene or death investigation, as well as a tribute to the skills and experience that make a competent forensic archaeologist; but also because it contains information useful to police officers, crime scene investigators, professional archaeologists starting to work in the forensic field, scientists and students. The potential of forensic archaeology cannot be underestimated.

References

Barber, M. 2011. *A History of Aerial Photography and Archaeology: Mata Hari's Glass Eye and Other Stories*. English Heritage, Swindon.

Blau, S. and Ubelaker, D. (eds) 2009. *Handbook of Forensic Anthropology and Archaeology*. Left Coast Press, Walnut Creek, CA.

Cheetham, P.N. and Hanson, I. 2009. Excavation and recovery in forensic archaeological investigations. In S. Blau and D. Ubelaker (eds) *Handbook of Forensic Anthropology and Archaeology*. Left Coast Press, Walnut Creek, California, pp. 141–149.

Connor, M.A. 2007. *Forensic Methods: Excavation for the Archaeologist and Investigator*. Altamira Press, Lanham, MD.

Cox, M. 2009. Forensic anthropology and archaeology: past and present – a United Kingdom perspective. In S. Blau and D. Ubelaker (eds) *Handbook of Forensic Anthropology and Archaeology*. Left Coast Press, Walnut Creek, CA, pp. 29–41.

Cox, M., Flavel, A., Hanson, I. *et al.* (eds) 2008. *The Scientific Investigation of Mass Graves. Towards Protocols and Standard Operating Procedures*. Cambridge University Press, Cambridge.

Dilley, R. 2005. Legal matters. In J. Hunter and M. Cox (eds) *Forensic Archaeology: Advances in Theory and Practice*. Routledge, London, pp. 177–203.

Dirkmaat, D.C. (ed.) 2012. *A Companion to Forensic Anthropology*. Blackwell Publishing Ltd, Oxford.

Dirkmaat, D.C., Cabo, L.C., Ousley, S.D. and Symes, S.A. 2008. New perspectives in forensic anthropology. *Yearbook of Physical Anthropology* 51: 33–52.

Dupras, T.L., Schultz, J.J., Wheeler, S.M. and Williams, L.J. 2006. *Forensic Recovery of Human Remains: Archaeological Approaches*. CRC Press, Boca Raton, FL.

Ferllini, R. 2007. *Forensic Archaeology and Human Rights Violations*. Charles C Thomas, Springfield, IL.

Haglund, W.D., Connor, M. and Scott, D.D. 2001. The archaeology of contemporary mass graves. *Historical Archaeology* 35: 57–69.

Hunter, J. 2009. Domestic homicide investigations in the United Kingdom. In S. Blau and D. Ubelaker (eds) *Handbook of Forensic Anthropology and Archaeology*. Left Coast Press, Walnut Creek, CA, pp. 363–373.

Hunter, J. and Cox, M. 2005. *Forensic Archaeology: Advances in Theory and Practice*. Routledge, London.

Hunter, J.R., Brickley, M.B., Bourgeois, J. *et al.* 2001. Forensic archaeology, forensic anthropology and human rights in Europe. *Science & Justice* 41: 173–178.

Hunter, J.R., Heron, C., Janaway, R.C. *et al.* 1994. Forensic archaeology in Britain. *Antiquity* 68: 758–769.

Killam, E.W. 2004. *The Detection of Human Remains*, 2nd edn. Charles C Thomas, Springfield, IL.

Márquez-Grant, N., Acinas Robledo, M.M. and Sánchez-Sánchez, J.A. 2011. El papel de la arqueología en la investigación criminal. *Revista de la Escuela de Medicina Legal* 16: 14–22.

Márquez-Grant, N., Litherland, S. and Roberts, J. 2012. European perspectives and the role of the forensic archaeologist in the UK. In D.C. Dirkmaat (ed.) *A Companion to Forensic Anthropology*. Blackwell Publishing Ltd, Oxford, pp. 598–625.

Owsley, D.W. 2001. Why the forensic anthropologist needs the archaeologist. *Historical Archaeology* **35**: 35–38.

Powers, N. and Sibun, L. (2011). *Standards and Guidance for Forensic Archaeologists*. Institute for Archaeologists, Reading.

Scott, D.D. and Connor, M. 2001. The role and future of archaeology in forensic science, *Historical Archaeology* **35**: 101–104.

Servello, J.A. 2010. *Thermal Identification of Clandestine Burials: A Signature Analysis and Image Classification Approach. Denton, Texas. UNT Digital Library*. http://digital.library.unt.edu/ark:/67531/metadc33201/ (accessed 20 January 2012).

Tuller, H. and Djurić, M. 2006. Keeping the pieces together: comparison of mass grave excavation methodology, *Forensic Science International* **156**: 192–200.

Appendix 3.1 CONTEXT RECORDING FORM
(adapted and modified from: Museum of London Archaeology Service,1994 (3rd edn). *Archaeology Site Manual*. Museum of London, London)

SITE NAME	OPERATION	FORCE	CFS CASE NO.	CONTEXT NO.

CONTEXT TYPE				
deposit	fill	layer	cut	structure

DEPOSIT	ARBITRARY LAYER – describe as deposit – CLEANING LAYER	CUT
1. **Composition**		1. **Shape in plan**
		2. **Corners**
2. **Colour**		3. **Size** (l, b, d)
		4. **Slope break Top**
3. **Composition/** particle size (+10%)		5. **Sides**
		6. **Base**
4. **Inclusions** (−10%)		7. **Profile**
		8. **Orientation**
5. **Extent** (length, breadth, depth)		9. **Truncation**
		10. **Fill nos**
Other comments, method and conditions		**Other comments**

RELATIONSHIPS (stratigraphic not physical)	(deposit or type of layer, **cut or other feature**)
Earlier than	(below, sealed by, **cut by, filled by**)
Contemporary	(with, equivalent to, **same as**)
Later than	(above, seals, fill of, **cuts**)

EVIDENCE (number, originator and type)	RECORDING (number, originator and type)
Environmental	Plan
Artefactual	Section
Sieving	Photography
Metal detection/other	Site note book/other

INTERPRETATION

Date_____

Recorded by_____

Signature_____

Checked by_____

Appendix 3.1 CONTEXT RECORDING FORM

(adapted and modified from: Museum of London Archaeology Service,1994 (3rd edn). *Archaeology Site Manual.* Museum of London, London)

SITE NAME	OPERATION	FORCE	CFS CASE NO.	CONTEXT NO.

SKETCH PLAN or PROFILE (give approx. scale, orientation)

Other notes

Date_____

Recorded by_____

Signature_____

Checked by_____

4

Forensic anthropology

Julie Roberts[1] and Nicholas Márquez-Grant[2]
[1]*Cellmark Forensic Services, Chorley, UK*
[2]*Cellmark Forensic Services, Abingdon, UK; and Institute of Human Sciences, School of Anthropology and Museum Ethnography, University of Oxford, Oxford, UK*

4.1 Introduction

This chapter discusses the role of the Forensic Anthropologist at the crime scene and in the mortuary and provides guidelines on the appropriate protocols to follow. It does not describe technical methods in detail as there are already many good reference texts available that fulfil this requirement (Komar and Buikstra, 2008; Schmitt *et al.*, 2006; Byers, 2005; Krogman and İşcan, 1986; Cox and Mays, 2000; Stewart, 1979; Blau and Ubelaker, 2009; Bass, 2005). The procedures employed by anthropologists in disaster victim identification (DVI), and the excavation and examination of individuals from mass graves are also well documented by other authors (Cox *et al.*, 2008; Black *et al.*, 2010a; Jensen, 2000; Haglund and Sorg, 2002; Ferllini, 2003). Whilst reference is made to mass fatality incidents, the primary focus of this chapter is to provide police officers and CSIs who may wish to use the services of an anthropologist, with an awareness of how this particular area of expertise might assist them in their criminal investigations. It also aims to provide trainee forensic anthropologists and students with an introduction to standard anthropological procedures from the first call to a crime scene through to the mortuary and finally to the production of an expert witness statement for use in court.

4.2 The role of the Forensic Anthropologist in criminal investigation

Forensic anthropology can be defined as the application of methods and principles of physical anthropology (the study of humans from the point of view of biology and

Forensic Ecology Handbook: From Crime Scene to Court, First Edition.
Edited by Nicholas Márquez-Grant and Julie Roberts.

physical characteristics), to cases of medico-legal or forensic interest. These skills may equally be utilised in humanitarian missions where authorities are seeking to establish the identity of the deceased, but not pursue a prosecution. The American Academy of Forensic Sciences defines forensic anthropology as the application of the science of physical or biological anthropology to the legal process or of cases of medico-legal significance, primarily by focusing on human skeletal or badly decomposed remains.

In the United Kingdom, the qualification and training undertaken to become a forensic anthropologist is usually separate from that required to become a foren- sic archaeologist (Hunter, 2002: xxv). The situation in the United States, where the discipline has a much longer and well-established history, is different. There, practitioners in forensic anthropology are dual trained in archaeology and routinely act as recovery team leaders taking responsibility for all aspects of archaeologi- cal excavation as well as analysis of remains (Hunter, 2002: xxv; Simmons and Haglund, 2005: 159; Burns 2007: 272; Heussner and Holland, 1999; Komar and Buikstra, 2008; Dirkmaat et al., 2008). In Spain, by contrast, the only people who can work as forensic anthropologists for the courts are usually medically trained and generally based in a governmental Medico-Legal Institute (Prieto, 2009). Thus, differences can be found between countries with regard to training and professional practice in forensic anthropology (for a review see Kranioti and Paine, 2011).

In practical terms, the forensic anthropologist applies standard scientific tech- niques developed in physical anthropology to the analysis of human remains that are unrecognisable (Simmons and Haglund, 2005: 159). This is usually for the purpose of assisting in the identification of the deceased. Human remains may be unidenti- fiable for a wide variety of reasons including natural decomposition, modification by fire and explosions, animals or even other humans. In these instances the an- thropologist will not only be able to provide information relating to the identity of the deceased, such as estimated age-at-death, sex, ancestry and stature where pos- sible, but he or she may also be able to comment on ante-mortem or post-mortem changes which may be relevant to the criminal investigation. For example, it will be possible to determine whether human remains were deliberately dismembered or whether disarticulation occurred as a result of natural processes or animal ac- tivity. Likewise, the experienced forensic anthropologist will be able to distinguish between fractures caused by traumatic injury and those caused by thermal damage in fatal fires.

At suspected or actual crime scenes, the forensic anthropologist will assist by locating and recovering human skeletal remains. He or she will often work in con- junction with a forensic archaeologist, botanist and entomologist, looking for such things as evidence of decomposition in situ, or plants and insects associated with the remains which might provide vital information about post-mortem interval (time- since-death). In the mortuary, the forensic anthropologist is largely concerned with providing biological data which will help to determine the identity of the deceased but he or she will also assist with trauma analysis. The specific functions of the anthropologist at the scene and in the mortuary will be discussed in more detail in Sections 4.4 and 4.5.

Most of the time the anthropologist will be working on cases relating to single individuals including unexplained and suspicious deaths, suicides and accidental deaths. However, he or she may also be asked to provide assistance in mass fatality incidents such as transportation accidents, war crimes, natural catastrophes, terrorist incidents or industrial accidents (Jensen, 2000: 115; Burns, 2007: 270; MacKinnon and Mundorff, 2006).

Anthropologists serving law enforcement agencies may be employed by universities, museums, or independent forensic service providers. They may also work as freelance consultants, or be based within police forces, governmental institutions and other organisations such as repatriation companies. In the sphere of war crimes investigations the anthropologist will most likely be working for national or international government agencies such as the Foreign and Commonwealth Office or the United Nations, or non-governmental organisations (NGOs) such as Physicians for Human Rights (PHR) or the Centre for International Forensic Assistance (CIFA). When dealing with multiple fatality incidents the anthropologist will most frequently be part of a multinational team such as the International Criminal Tribunal for Former Yugoslavia (ICTY) or the International Commission for Missing Persons (ICMP), or they may belong to a national team such as the Argentine Forensic Anthropology Team (EAAF) or the Disaster Mortuary Operational Response Team (DMORT) which operates throughout the United States (Burns, 2007: 277).

In the United States there are just over 80 diplomates of the American Board of Forensic Anthropology (http://www.theabfa.org/diplomates.html), although the number of practising forensic anthropologists is higher. Steadman and Haglund (2005) undertook a comprehensive study into the scope of anthropological contributions in human rights investigations. In it they considered the number of anthropologists deployed in the period 1990–1999, their nationalities, who they were employed by, their levels of education and qualifications, and the specific roles that they undertook. They identified that since 1990 the four largest organisations working in the field to investigate human rights atrocities (EAAF, FAFG, PHR and ICTY) had deployed 'a minimum of 134 anthropologists and archaeologists of 22 different nationalities to 33 different countries' (Steadman and Haglund, 2005: 7). Steadman and Haglund found that duties included exhumations (the most frequent task that anthropologists were involved in), skeletal analysis, seminars and training, logistics and assessment of ante-mortem data. Quite often the primary aim of the mission might start as one thing and end as another, as in the Balkans where forensic anthropologists were initially employed by various organisations to produce information that could be used by the criminal tribunal in The Hague, and subsequently became engaged in long-term humanitarian projects to identify the deceased under the auspices of the ICMP.

The core skills of the forensic anthropologist relate to species (human vs non-human) and fragment identification, victim identification (biological profile), trauma analysis and analysis of ante-mortem or post-mortem modifications. More specialised areas of forensic anthropology include assessment of age in living individuals through the examination of radiographs (Black *et al.*, 2010b), analysis and interpretation of burnt remains (Schmidt and Symes, 2008), facial analysis and reconstruction (Wilkinson, 2004), and gait analysis (Lynnerup and Vedel, 2005) amongst other areas (see Thompson and Black, 2006).

In addition to practising their own expertise, the anthropologist should be competent in advising CSIs and police officers on other related scientific techniques such as the dating of bone (Chapter 7) and the potential for DNA or isotope analysis (Chapters 6 and 7 respectively). He or she should be aware of which samples to take for specialist analysis and how to take them at the post-mortem examination.

In the United Kingdom, it is *not* the responsibility of the forensic anthropologist to determine or certify the cause of death. This is the remit of the forensic pathologist alone. The anthropologist may assist with this, however, by distinguishing between ante-mortem and post-mortem trauma and modification, and the physical reconstruction of fragmented remains which allows the forensic pathologist to observe more clearly any skeletal defects such as gunshot wounds.

4.3   Pre-scene attendance

In the United Kingdom, a request for assistance at the scene or in the mortuary is likely to come from a CSM or Senior CSI, a Forensic Coordinator, or a Senior Investigating Officer (SIO). When the anthropologist receives such a call, it is important that he or she records the time and date of the conversation, the name of the person calling and the police force they belong to, and summarises the request and subsequent discussions. These contemporaneous notes are disclosable in court therefore it is important that they are both comprehensive and legible. If it is not volunteered by the officer on the telephone, the anthropologist should request the following information:

- Background to the case, including the date of discovery of the remains.

- The circumstances surrounding the discovery, including whether they were disturbed at the time of or following discovery.

- The condition and state of preservation of the remains.

- The environmental context in which they were found.

- The location of the scene and contact details of the person they will be meeting.

Prior to attending the scene the anthropologist should formulate a preliminary strategy based on the information given, although this will almost inevitably have to be adapted on arrival at the scene. Health and safety should also be considered and a risk assessment completed but that too, by necessity, will be dynamic.

The anthropologist should work on the principle that he or she will need to provide all the equipment necessary for the recovery and recording of human remains at the scene. As the post-mortem examination will often take place immediately after the remains are recovered, equipment for the mortuary should also be taken. Below is a list of the equipment that will be required:

- Protective personal equipment (PPE) including scene suits, gloves, masks, hairnets and overshoes.

- Tools for excavating and recording the remains and deposition or burial site. These should include a spade, shovel, trowels, fine hand tools such as a 'plasterers leaf', measuring tapes (at least one 30 m tape as well as 5 and 8 m tapes, sieves, brushes, buckets and drawing equipment (see also Chapter 3).

- Mortuary equipment including digital and dial callipers, osteometric board, measuring tape, pubic symphysis and rib end morphology reference casts.

- Equipment to take DNA samples including sterile blades and scalpels, tweezers and universal pots (these may be provided by the mortuary but it is best to be prepared).

- Appropriate reference texts, for example formulae for calculation of estimated stature.

- Skeletal recording forms. These may vary from organisation to organisation but should all contain sections relating to the following:

  - taphonomy, bones present and absent, estimation of ancestry, age at death, sex, stature, bone morphology, metric data, trauma and other skeletal pathology, unique identifying features.

4.4 Scene attendance

The time of arrival at (and departure from) the scene should be documented, as should the presence of all other personnel in attendance. It is usual for the anthropologist to receive a briefing at the local police station or outside the scene (if they have arranged to go directly there) prior to entering the inner cordon. This provides the opportunity to discuss the strategy with the CSM and SIO (if present). This discussion should include a consideration of the needs of other specialists as well as CSIs and PolSAs. It is always good to have an initial walk through the scene, via the common approach path, with the CSM prior to commencing specialist work. This helps the specialist to become familiar with the landscape and ask any additional questions once the remains have been viewed in context.

At the scene, the skeletonised or decomposed remains may be lying on the surface in an articulated or disarticulated state and possibly spread over a wide area so that an element of search may be required. If the remains are articulated and partially or fully buried, the police may already have requested the attendance of an archaeologist (see Chapter 3).

The first priority of the anthropologist will be to confirm whether the remains that have been discovered are human or not, although the possibility of them being non-human may already have been eliminated by examination of images sent electronically prior to attendance at the scene. If the remains do prove to be human the next priority is to determine whether they are ancient or modern in date and of interest to the police. This can be established at the scene by a number of means including assessment of any associated clothing, documentation or personal effects, the condition of the bones, the presence of any modern dental work, and burial or deposition context. Quite often it is a combination of these things which will determine whether the remains are deemed of forensic or medico-legal interest. Whether the remains are designated archaeological or modern is highly dependent on the country in which they are found, as this can vary greatly according to national law (see Márquez-Grant and Fibiger, 2011).

With regard to burial and deposition contexts, the services of an archaeologist will almost certainly be required unless the anthropologist is dually qualified. The anthropologist should also provide advice regarding the attendance of other specialists at the scene, for example botanists and entomologists.

Once an initial assessment of the scene has been made, the anthropologist should then assist in formulating a strategy for recording and recovering the remains for post-mortem examination. This should include a consideration of whether they have decomposed *in situ* or whether they have been dumped or buried there some time after death when the decomposition process has already begun. A degree of disturbance and cross-contamination of the scene is inevitable as a result of the remains being discovered in the first place; however, prior to any more activity taking place, the anthropologist should, at this point, be considering the collection of pollen and soil samples which could potentially be used to link a suspect to the scene (see Chapters 10 and 12).

All photography at the scene will be undertaken by a CSI or forensic photographer (see Chapter 14) but advice should be given by the anthropologist regarding any detailed images of the remains or surrounding vegetation and insects that are required.

Several methods can be used to record and recover surface remains and the anthropologist will make a judgement as to which are most appropriate for that particular scene (Figure 4.1). For scenes where bones or body parts are scattered over a large area it is best practice to create a grid or divide the area into zones depending on the terrain. As well as facilitating systematic and complete recovery of all skeletal elements at the scene, these methods provide a basis for the accurate location and recording of evidence. Further techniques for recording human remains at crime scenes, which are beyond the scope of the present chapter, can be found elsewhere in the literature (e.g. Dupras *et al.*, 2012; Fairgrieve, 2008; Dirkmaat, 2012).

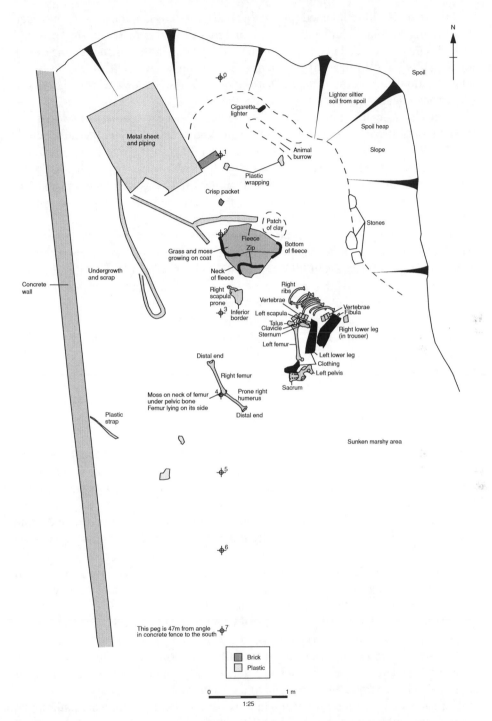

Figure 4.1 Surface deposition in a forensic case. The anthropologist plotted the location of the remains, identified the bones and drew their correct orientation. Courtesy of Cellmark Forensic Services. Illustration by Georgina Slater.

If the body is still articulated (joined together by soft tissue) the position in which it is laying, including orientation and individual positions of the head, arms and legs, should be recorded in detail. This may be of value in reconstructing the events immediately prior to death if the victim died at the scene, or it may help in the interpretation of the circumstances surrounding deposition or burial if the victim was already dead when they were brought there.

In all cases, legible notes should be augmented with photographs (with scale and/or North arrow where appropriate), plans and sketches. Planning may be undertaken by specialist police support units depending on the size and complexity of the scene and the resources of the police force involved. It is still important, however, that the anthropologist makes his or her own measured sketch plans. The position of the remains relative to other key features and significant evidence within the scene should also be noted and planned or sketched.

Once recovery is complete and the scene and recovery process have been properly documented, the anthropologist should be able to compile an inventory of the bones/body parts present and inform the CSM of any missing elements, although a detailed assessment of this may have to wait until examination in the mortuary depending on the level of disruption and dispersal of the remains. It may also be possible to provide the CSM or SIO with a preliminary assessment of whether the deceased is adult or non-adult, male or female, and to comment on any obvious traumatic injury, although detailed conclusions should be reserved until after the post-mortem examination is complete.

4.5   In the mortuary

When working in the mortuary it is important that the forensic anthropologist engages with the mortuary manager or technician prior to commencing the examination in order to familiarise him or herself with the layout of the mortuary, the facilities available and health and safety policies. Key points to clarify include where the clean and dirty areas are within the building, the correct route in and out of the post-mortem examination room (usually this is via a changing room), the location of scrubs and mortuary PPE, which sink to use when remains are covered in soil or decomposed soft tissue (the post-mortem room will generally have a designated sink with a soil trap for washing these), macerating facilities for flesh-covered remains, and procedures for disposal of clinical waste.

As at the scene, the anthropologist should document the location of the mortuary, the start and finish time of the post-mortem examination, and a list of the names and roles of people present at the examination. The Operation name and/or Police reference number, laboratory reference number, date and signature of the anthropologist should also be recorded on every page of any contemporaneous notes.

The forensic post-mortem examination is usually led by a forensic pathologist (in the United Kingdom, he or she will be Home Office registered). It is always advisable to discuss with the pathologist prior to commencing the examination, how he or she wishes to proceed with regard to the anthropological input. The forensic

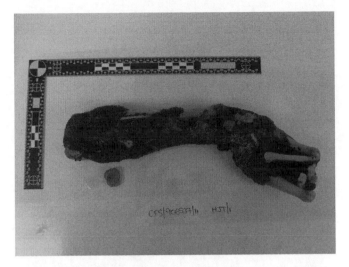

Figure 4.2 This 'body part' was submitted to the DNA laboratory as police thought it to be a human arm. On inspection by an anthropologist it was confirmed as non-human (it was in fact a seal limb). Courtesy of Cellmark Forensic Services. (To see a colour version of this figure, please see Plate 4.2.)

pathologist or SIO may also have requested the presence of other specialists, such as an odontologist, entomologist or ballistics expert, and a strategy and sequence of examination will be discussed between all involved. The anthropologist should not remove any clothing or soft tissue unless requested to do so by the forensic pathologist.

Where remains are extensively decomposed or skeletonised, the anthropologist will initially be engaged in processing them, that is for example, cleaning them in warm water and a mild surfactant, and laying them out on the examination table in the correct anatomical alignment. Once this has been achieved, working closely with the pathologist, he or she will seek to undertake the following:

Eliminate any bones that are non-human. The anthropologist should be able, from macroscopic examination, to identify the remains as human or non-human (Figure 4.2) and to remove any incidental non-human bone that may have been collected by police search teams, for example. Where species cannot be determined due to high levels of fragmentation, this should be recorded and further microscopic, histological or biomolecular analysis recommended as appropriate (see Chapter 7).

Identify the skeletal elements (bones) present. The anthropologist should have a thorough knowledge of human skeletal anatomy and should be able to identify fragments to a particular element or category of bone (Figure 4.3). He or she should also be familiar with the appearance of ossified cartilaginous tissue (cartilage that has turned to bone because of the aging process or underlying pathology), as well as the normal variations that can occur within the human skeleton such as additional vertebrae and cervical ribs.

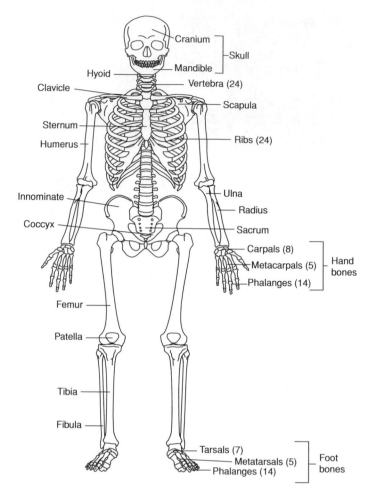

Figure 4.3   Chart of the human skeleton showing some basic skeletal terminology. The average adult human skeleton is composed of 206 bones (in addition to teeth).

Compile an inventory. Once the bones have been identified and reassembled in anatomical position, the anthropologist will compile a detailed inventory of the bones, recording which ones are present, which ones are missing, and noting any damaged or missing parts. An inventory of the dentition may be completed by the anthropologist but if odontology is to be used as a means of identification (see Bowers, 2010), particularly if the matching of ante-mortem and post-mortem dental records is required, then the opinion of a forensic odontologist is essential.

Comment on state of preservation and taphonomy (the study of factors affecting the body between death and discovery). An assessment of the condition of the remains will assist in determining post-mortem interval. In addition, information on bone modification such as burning, weathering, or scavenging marks may prove valuable to the interpretation of circumstances surrounding death or provide an indication of what happened to the body between death and discovery.

Record the number of individuals present. The anthropologist will establish whether there are any repeated skeletal elements, for example two left femora (thigh bones) or elements that are not repeated but have clearly come from individuals of different age and sex, for instance an adult left femur and a juvenile right humerus (arm bone). Where non-diagnostic and non-repeated fragments are present which cannot be categorically designated as coming from separate individuals, this can only be expressed as a *minimum* number, referred to as the Minimum Number of Individuals (MNI). The 'Most Likely Number of Individuals' (MLNI) is a calculation which has also been used (Adams and Konigsberg, 2004, 2008) and this is self-explanatory, but it is not always common practice to express the numbers of individuals in commingled and fragmented remains in this way. If there is more than one individual present in an assemblage of disarticulated bone, the anthropologist will attempt to group the elements according to individual, also providing any additional anthropological data that might help to establish identity. Ultimately, a decision will be made by the pathologist, the anthropologist and the police regarding which of the elements should be submitted for DNA analysis to confirm identity.

Reconstruct fragmented remains. It may be necessary to physically reconstruct fragmented remains in order to undertake facial analysis or examine specific fracture patterns. Where remains are still wet, one of the most commonly used glues in mortuaries is 'Zap-A-Gap®' in conjunction with 'Zip Kicker™' accelerant. The use of these two solutions together creates a thermal reaction which can generate a lot of heat and form a permanent bond within seconds. It requires manual dexterity and practice to work with these mediums as it is easy for gloves to inadvertently become stuck to the bone and the anthropologist must be absolutely certain that the fragments they are joining do actually match before they commit! Speaking from personal experience it is extremely difficult to un-stick fragments joined by this glue even using 100 % acetone. If the anthropologist is less confident and the remains are dry, water-soluble glue may be used instead as this is easier to remove.

Trauma analysis. The anthropologist should be able to make an assessment of whether any breaks in the bone were caused before, after or around the time of death. It can be particularly difficult to distinguish between trauma sustained immediately before and immediately after death – damage which is often termed 'peri-mortem trauma'. This is because bone which is still flesh-covered and moist will react in largely the same way to mechanical forces applied to it, whether the person is dead or alive (Haglund and Sorg, 2002; Byres, 2005). It is only once the body decomposes and the bones lose moisture that they will break in a different way (Haglund and Sorg, 2002; Byres, 2005). Generally speaking it is the location and characteristics of lesions that make them diagnostic of ante-mortem trauma and specific injury types. These might include gunshot wounds, sharp and blunt force trauma and explosive injuries (Clark, 1999; Lewis and Rutty, 2003; Galloway, 1999; Galloway *et al.*, 1999; Di Maio, 1999; Kimmerle and Baraybar, 2008; Berryman and Symes, 1995). Ultimately it is the responsibility of the pathologist to provide a final opinion on any traumatic injury present, although depending on his or her level of experience he or she might be less familiar than the anthropologist with post-mortem fracture patterns in decomposed and skeletonised remains.

Victim identification. The anthropologist will be very familiar with all current techniques relating to estimation of age-at-death, ancestry, sex, stature, body build and individuating features. He or she will be aware of the accuracy and limitations of each method and also factors that cause variations to the norm. For example, ossification (turning to bone) of the costal cartilage can occur prematurely in heroin addicts and arthritis can develop at the ends of the ribs and the sternum (Molle *et al.*, 1984; Gifford *et al.*, 1975; Brancos *et al.*, 1991). If the anthropologist is not aware of this then an older age can be wrongly assigned.

At the end of an examination, depending on the condition and completeness of the remains, the anthropologist should be able to provide the SIO with a realistic estimate of how old the individual was when they died (presented as an age range and not a single value), whether they were male or female, their ancestry, stature and a record of previous injuries and any medical conditions such as arthritis, specific and non-specific infections which had affected the bones. This information constitutes what is termed a 'biological profile' which is in essence a summary of the physical characteristics of the deceased when they were last alive. Where possible anthropological data, particularly old injuries and individuating features, should be presented to the SIO in terms of how they would have appeared in the living individual. For example, a badly healed compound fracture and shortening of the left tibia would have meant that the deceased may have walked with a pronounced limp on their left side, or a healed, displaced fracture to the nasal bones might have meant a bent and twisted nose in life. The purpose of this is to try and make the victim recognisable to family and friends and also to allow for a comparison to be made with any information of that type held on the Missing Persons Database or local missing persons lists.

Whilst it is hoped that the anthropologist will be able to provide an opinion of post-mortem interval and a comprehensive set of biological data that will assist in the identification of the deceased, it should be pointed out that this is not always achievable. If the remains are in a particularly poor condition, if the body is incomplete, or if the deceased is represented by only a few fragments of bone, it will sometimes only be possible to provide the most basic information (Komar and Potter, 2007).

4.6   Positive identification

Together with the odontologist, the forensic anthropologist is often the 'front-line' in terms of identification of the deceased and in some countries these disciplines alone are used to confirm identity. In the United Kingdom, this is not the case and the Coroner or Procurator Fiscal almost always stipulates that identity must be confirmed by DNA profiling (see Chapter 6). This brings some specific problems in relation to the identification of decomposed unrecognisable remains. In the

United Kingdom, British citizens are not required to register their DNA profile on the National DNA Database unless they have committed a criminal offence (or been cautioned for one). In many instances, therefore, even if it is possible to successfully obtain a full DNA profile from unidentified remains, a positive identity cannot be confirmed on the basis of this because there is nothing to compare it to. This problem is compounded if there is no clue as to the identity of the deceased and reference profiles cannot be obtained from family members for comparison. In other cases it may not be possible to obtain a profile from the deceased due to the degradation of soft tissue and bone, although this is becoming increasingly rare as new techniques in DNA analysis are continually being developed (see Chapter 6).

In cases such as those described above, anthropology can be used to narrow down the parameters relating to the biological profile of the deceased and this information can then act as a starting point in the identification process, enabling family liaison officers to approach families who have missing relatives who broadly fit the description given. Additional information can be provided by anthropologists specialized in facial reconstruction (e.g. Wilkinson, 2004; Taylor, 2000) who can create a model or an image of how the person may have looked when they were alive.

The extraction of DNA from burnt remains where all organic matter has been combusted continues to be a problem but unless there is extensive fragmentation of the bone, anthropological methods can still be used to assess such things as age-at-death and skeletal pathology.

4.7   Production of an Expert Witness Statement and court attendance

The forensic anthropologist is required not only to undertake the examination of human remains but to present his or her findings in a formal statement or report. In England and Wales, this statement may then be used by the police, the CPS, the Coroner, defence lawyers and, perhaps most importantly of all, the jury (Rothwell, 2004). The anthropologist may then be ordered to appear as an expert witness in a coroner's or criminal court to present and defend the evidence in their statement, or the statement may just be accepted without the anthropologist being cited to attend (Ranson, 2009; Henneberg, 2008, 2009).

The key points to remember in relation to this are that the statement must be understandable to a person with no scientific background, that the specialist is confident of any conclusions arrived at and can back them up with evidence, facts and published references, and that he or she does not step outside the limits of his or her expertise.

With regard to the court appearance itself, the anthropologist must be confident, professional in appearance and manner, and able to communicate well and clearly. It is also important to remember that any questioning of scientific findings is not a personal attack (although sometimes it may feel like it) and it is vital that the expert witness remains calm and logical during cross-examination. The evidence might be of the highest quality, but this is of no use whatsoever if the anthropologist delivering and defending it appears uncertain, flustered, or allows his or herself to be drawn into a discussion that falls outside their sphere of expertise. Maintaining credibility in the eyes of the court and particularly the jury is of paramount importance.

Anthropologists in the United Kingdom do not automatically receive expert witness training and this is a serious omission which needs to be addressed. Some university courses do include this as part of their degree programmes, but forensic anthropology degrees are a relatively new phenomenon and there are many experienced practitioners who undertook anatomy or archaeology degrees as a means of embarking on their career, which did not include this element. This can, and should, be rectified by continuous professional development and attendance on expert witness courses, such as the widely recognised one offered by the legal training consultancy, Bond Solon (www.bondsolon.com). Forensic anthropologists working for independent forensic service providers may also be offered expert witness training by the organisation that employs them.

As well as being written clearly and in a manner that can be understood by persons with a non-scientific and medical background, a good witness statement should include the following sections:

1. A heading which includes the CJ Act and Criminal Procedure Rules (in England and Wales), the name and qualifications of the person writing the statement, the organisation they work for, a statement relating to the integrity of their evidence and a date and signature. An example of this is provided below:

Witness Statement

(CJ Act 1967, s 9 MC Act, 1980, ss 5A (3a), and 5B Criminal Procedure Rules, 2005, r 27)

Statement of	Julie Ann Roberts, BA (Hons), MSc, PhD
Age	Over 18
Occupation	Forensic Anthropologist and Archaeologist
	At
	Cellmark Forensic Services
	16 Blacklands Way, Abingdon Business Park, Abingdon, Oxfordshire, OX14 1DY

This statement consisting of 15 pages each signed by me, is true to the best of my knowledge and belief and I make it known that, if it is tendered in evidence, I shall be liable to prosecution if I have wilfully stated in it anything which I know to be false or do not believe to be true.

Dated the 7th Day of January 2012

Signature. . . . .

2. The Police Operation Name and Reference Number
   This will be designated by the police force and should be cross-referenced to the anthropologist's laboratory reference number.

3. A short summary of the qualifications and experience of the anthropologist.

4. Background information
   This would include the immediate circumstances surrounding the case and the discovery of the remains. This information is usually obtained from a briefing delivered by the police and that provided on any forensic submission form.

5. The work request
   This should include details of who requested the work, when it was requested and what was agreed between the anthropologist and the CSM, SIO or Forensic Coordinator.

6. Scene and/or mortuary attendance
   As described above this will include locations visited, dates and times of arrival and departure, other personnel present and their roles.

7. Methods used
   This may also be described as 'nature of examination'. The methods used at the scene and in the mortuary or laboratory should be described and fully referenced. Details of any statistical analysis should also be provided here.

8. Results of the examination
   This should detail in full the findings from the examinations and include summary analytical and metric data. Long lists of numerical data, calculations and inventories of highly fragmented material (for example burnt bone) should be contained within an appendix, and referred to in the results section. This makes the findings of the anthropologist more accessible to the jury whilst still allowing them to see any raw data that might be significant.

9. Conclusions
   The conclusions should summarise the results and include an interpretation of them. Findings relating to most 'traditional' forensic evidence types, such as fibres or body fluids will be expressed in terms of strength of evidence. This may be difficult to achieve with regard to anthropological analysis but it may still be possible to use similar terminology with which the courts are familiar. For example, the primary question being asked by the police might be, whether the skeletal development of a child was consistent with normal development for his or her chronological age. If the anthropologist finds that skeletal development was considerably delayed, he or she might say that the evidence relating to this strongly supports the conclusion that the child's skeleton was not developing at a normal rate. If the anthropologist also identified the presence of Harris lines (indicating periods of arrested growth) on the bones together with evidence of pathology associated with nutritional disorders, he or she might then go on to

make inferences regarding the health and nutritional status of the child. At this point recommendations for further analysis or the opinions of other specialists might also be made.

10. References, Appendices and Technical Notes
Full references of any texts referred to in the statement should be listed. Appendices should contain the details of any assistants used during the course of the examinations, and lists of exhibits received and created (with details of transfers between police officers and laboratories). Diagrams and glossaries for reference purposes and tables of results may also be included here. It is good practice to include a Technical Note in the main body of the statement which refers to the location of the case file and any related archived material such as images and medical notes. It should also be acknowledged that these items can be disclosed in full providing sufficient notice is given.

4.8 Conclusion

There has been an upsurge in the use of forensic anthropology in recent years. Further training institutions have been created, more research programmes and new techniques are being developed as can be observed from publications in journals such as *Journal of Forensic Science* and *Forensic Science International*. Increasing awareness through training and seminars and other events have highlighted the vital role of the forensic anthropologist in death scene investigation where the remains are in an advanced state of decomposition, burnt or dismembered, or skeletonised. This is not to forget advances made in the application of skills to the living as well as the dead, in areas such as age estimation where radiographs are taken of some individuals to estimate their true chronological age as much as possible (e.g. Schmeling *et al.*, 2008; Black *et al.*, 2010b).

Historically and currently, forensic anthropologists have worked in a variety of scenarios, some focusing on individual police cases and some working primarily on humanitarian missions and mass fatality incidents. Some are researchers dedicating themselves to developing important methods that will provide more precision in current techniques, for example increased accuracy for age-at-death estimation. Forensic anthropologists can also play an influential role in some aspects of society, be it the recovery and identification of victims of the Spanish Civil War and pressures to change legislation to promote the return of deceased to the families, by giving evidence in criminal cases or assisting in human rights work.

A balance between casework and research is necessary, where casework can generate research ideas which are directly relevant to criminal investigations and where research is required to assist with a case, for example in the estimation of postmortem interval or the effects of a saw cutting through a bone. New techniques and standards are increasingly being accepted in court (for example the *Daubert* criteria in the United States, see Komar and Buikstra, 2008). These methods must, however, be supported by credible research and used by practitioners who are competent in how to apply them and interpret the results. There is also a move towards presenting anthropological findings in a way that is more closely aligned to the 'traditional' forensic disciplines, for example using a Bayesian approach.

A number of countries in Europe and in other continents are at present creating national associations which are in turn setting up their own working groups to develop the field. In the United Kingdom, the British Association of Forensic Anthropology (BAFA) has a number of working groups and together with the Forensic Science Regulator, the discipline is seeking to obtain evidence of accreditation and competency amongst those practising members.

Ultimately, in crime scene investigation it is a multidisciplinary approach that works best and consultation between the anthropologist, CSM, SIO and Police Search Team leader at the beginning of a case can result in the best possible outcome for the job. By considering the questions asked of the anthropologist such as: How old are the remains? How many individuals are present? Who is the deceased? Can we reconstruct the events leading to death and deposition? and Can we identify any evidence linking to a third party?, expectations can be explored and clarified from the outset. It is anticipated that adopting this approach, together with future developments in methods, training and competency, will bring us closer to achieving our full potential as a discipline.

References

Adams, B.J. and Konigsberg, L.W. 2004. Estimation of the most likely number of individuals from commingled human skeletal remains. *American Journal of Physical Anthropology* **125**: 138–151.

Adams, B.J. and Konigsberg, L.W. 2008. How many people? Determining the number of individuals represented by commingled human remains. In B.J. Adams and J.E. Byrd (eds) *Recovery, Analysis, and Identification of Commingled Human Remains*. Humana Press, Totowa, NJ, pp. 241–256.

Bass, W.M. 2005. *Human Osteology: A Laboratory and Field Manual*, 5th edn. Missouri Archaeological Society No. 2, Columbia, MO.

Berryman, H.E. and Symes, S.A. 1995. Recognising gunshot and blunt cranial trauma through fracture interpretation. In K. Reichs (ed.) *Forensic Osteology: Advances in the Identification of Human Remains*, 2nd edn. Charles C Thomas, Springfield, IL, pp. 333–352.

Black, S.M., Walker, G., Hackman, L. and Brooks, C. (eds) 2010a. *Disaster Victim Identification: The Practitioner's Guide*. Dundee University Press, Dundee.

Black, S.M., Aggrawal, A. and Payne-James, J. 2010b. *Age Estimation in the Living*. John Wiley & Sons, Ltd, Chichester.

Blau, S. and Ubelaker, D.H. (eds) 2009. *Handbook of Forensic Anthropology and Archaeology*. Left Coast Press, Walnut Creek, CA.

Bowers, C.M. (ed.) 2010. *Forensic Dental Evidence: An Investigator's Handbook*. Academic Press, New York.

Brancós, M.A., Peris, P., Miró, J.M. *et al.* 1991. Septic arthritis in heroin addicts. *Seminars in Arthritis and Rheumatism* **21**: 81–87.

Burns, K.R. 2007. *Forensic Anthropology Training Manual*, 2nd edn. Pearson-Prentice Hall, Upper Saddle River, NJ.

Byers, S. 2005. *Introduction to Forensic Anthropology: A Textbook*, 2nd edn. Allyn and Bacon, Boston.

Clark, J. 1999. ICTY Operations in Bosnia-Herzegovina 1999 Season. Report of the Chief Pathologist Kevljani Grave Site. Unpublished report submitted to ICTY.

Cox, M. and Mays, S. (eds) 2000. *Human Osteology in Archaeology and Forensic Science*. Cambridge University Press, Cambridge.

Cox, M., Flavel, A., Hanson, I. *et al.* (eds) 2008. *The Scientific Investigation of Mass Graves: Towards Protocols and Standard Operating Procedures*. Cambridge University Press, Cambridge.

Di Maio, V.J.M. 1999. *Gunshot Wounds: Practical Aspects of Firearms, Ballistics, and Forensic Techniques*, 2nd edn. CRC Press, Boca Raton, FL.

Dirkmaat, D.C. (ed.) 2012. *A Companion to Forensic Anthropology*. Blackwell Publishing Ltd, Oxford.

Dirkmaat, D.C., Cabo, L.L., Ousley, S.D. and Symes, S.A. 2008. New perspectives in forensic anthropology. *Yearbook of Physical Anthropology* **51**: 33–52.

Dupras, T.L., Schultz, J.J., Wheller, S.M. and Williams, L.J. 2012. *Forensic Recovery of Human Remains: Archaeological Approaches*, 2nd edn. CRC Press/Taylor & Francis, Boca Raton, FL.

Fairgrieve, S.I. 2008. *Forensic Cremation: Recovery and Analysis*. CRC Press, Boca Raton, FL.

Ferllini, R. 2003. The development of human rights investigations since 1945. *Science and Justice Volume* **43**: 211–224.

Galloway, A. (ed.) 1999. *Broken Bones: Anthropological Analysis of Blunt Force Trauma*. Charles C Thomas, Springfield, IL.

Galloway, A., Symes, S.A, Haglund, W.D. and France, D.L. 1999. The role of forensic anthropology in trauma analysis. In A. Galloway (ed.) *Broken Bones: Anthropological Analysis of Blunt Force Trauma*. Charles C Thomas, Springfield, IL.

Gifford, D.B., Patzakis, M., Ivler, D. and Swezy, R.L. 1975. Septic arthritis due to pseudomonas in heroin addicts. *Journal of Bone and Joint Surgery, American Volume* **57**: 631–635.

Haglund, W.D. and Sorg, M.H. (eds) 2002. *Advances in Forensic Taphonomy: Method, Theory and Archaeological Perspectives*. CRC Press, Boca Raton, FL.

Henneberg, M. 2008. Expert Witness in a courtroom: Australian experience. In M. Oxenham (ed.) *Forensic Approaches to Death, Disaster and Abuse*. Australian Academic Press, Bowen Hills, Qld, pp. 307–318.

Henneberg, M. 2009. The Expert Witness and the Court of Law. In S. Blau and D.H. Ubelaker (eds) *Handbook of Forensic Anthropology and Archaeology*. Left Coast Press, Walnut Creek, CA, pp. 490–494.

Heussner, T. and Holland, T. 1999. Worldwide CILHI Mission to Bring Home Missing Heroes. *Quartermaster Professional Bulletin*, Summer 1999. Available at: http://qmmuseum .lee.army.mil/mortuary/worldwide_cilhi_mission.htm (accessed 29 July 2007).

Hunter, J.R. 2002. Foreword: A pilgrim in forensic archaeology – A personal view. In W.D. Haglund and M.H. Sorg (eds) *Advances in Forensic Taphonomy: Method, Theory and Archaeological Perspectives*. CRC Press, Boca Raton, FL, pp. xxv–xxxi.

Jensen, R.A. 2000. *Mass Fatality and Casualty Incidents: A Field Guide*. CRC Press, Boca Raton, FL.

Kimmerle, E.H. and Baraybar, J.P. 2008. *Skeletal Trauma: Identification of Injuries Resulting from Human Rights Abuse and Armed Conflict*. CRC Press/Taylor & Francis, Boca Raton, FL.

Komar, D. and Buikstra, J. 2008. *Forensic Anthropology: Contemporary Theory and Practice*. Oxford University Press, New York.

Komar, D. and Potter, W.E. 2007. Percentage of body recovered and its effect on identification rates and cause and manner of death determination. *Journal of Forensic Sciences* **52**: 528–531.

Kranioti, E. and Paine, R. 2011. Forensic anthropology in Europe: an assessment of current status and applications. *Journal of Anthropological Science* **89**: 71–92.

Krogman, W.M. and İşcan, M.Y. 1986. *The Human Skeleton in Forensic Medicine*. Charles C Thomas, Springfield, IL.

Lewis, M.E. and Rutty, G.N. 2003. The endangered child: the personal identification of children in forensic anthropology. *Science and Justice* **43**: 201–209.

Lynnerup, N. and Vedel, J. 2005. Person identification by gait analysis and photogrammetry. *Journal of Forensic Sciences* **50**: 112–118.

MacKinnon, G. and Mundorff, A.Z. 2006. The World Trade Center – September 11th 2001. In T. Thompson and S. Black (eds) *Forensic Human Identification: An Introduction*. CRC Press/Taylor & Francis, Boca Raton, FL, pp. 485–499.

Márquez-Grant, N. and Fibiger, L. 2011. *The Routledge Handbook of Archaeological Human Remains and Legislation: An International Guide to Laws and Practice in the Excavation and Treatment of Archaeological Human Remains*. Routledge, London.

Molle, D., Bard, H., Delphine, G. and Caquet, R. 1984. Sterno-chondro-costal joint arthritis in heroin addicts. Value of computed X-ray tomography. Four cases. *La Presse Médicale* **13**: 549–551. [in French]

Prieto, J.L. 2009. A history of forensic anthropology in Spain. In S. Blau and D.H. Ubelaker (eds) *Handbook of Forensic Anthropology and Archaeology*. Left Coast Press, Walnut Creek, CA, pp. 56–66.

Ranson, D. 2009. Legal aspects of identification. In S. Blau and D.H. Ubelaker (eds) *Handbook of Forensic Anthropology and Archaeology*. Left Coast Press, Walnut Creek, CA, pp. 495–508.

Rothwell, T. 2004. Presentation of Expert Forensic Evidence. In. P.C. White (ed.) *Crime Scene to Court: The Essentials of Forensic Science*, 2nd edn. Royal Society of Chemistry, London, pp. 414–439.

Schmeling, A., Grundmann, C., Furhmann, A. *et al.* 2008. Criteria for age estimation in living individuals. *International Journal of Legal Medicine* **122**: 457–460.

Schmidt, C.W. and Symes, S.A. (eds) 2008. *The Analysis of Burned Human Remains*. Academic Press/Elsevier, New York.

Schmitt, A., Cunha, E. and Pinheiro, E. (eds) 2006. *Forensic Anthropology and Medicine: Complementary Sciences from Recovery to Cause of Death*. Humana Press, Totowa, NJ.

Simmons, T. and Haglund, W.D. 2005. Anthropology in a forensic context. In J. Hunter and M. Cox (eds) *Forensic Archaeology: Advances in Theory and Practice*. Routledge, London, pp. 159–176.

Steadman, D.W. and Haglund, W.D. 2005. The scope of anthropological contributions to Human Rights Investigations. *Journal of Forensic Science* **50**: 1–8.

Stewart, T.D. 1979. *Essentials of Forensic Anthropology, Especially as Developed in the United States*. Charles C Thomas, Springfield, IL.

Taylor, K.T. 2000. *Forensic Art and Illustration*. CRC Press, Boca Raton, FL.

Thompson, T. and Black, S. (eds) 2006. *Forensic Human Identification: An Introduction*. CRC Press/Taylor & Francis, Boca Raton, FL.

Wilkinson, C.M. 2004. *Forensic Facial Reconstruction*. Cambridge University Press, Cambridge.

5

Forensic radiography

Mark Viner

Inforce Foundation, Cranfield Forensic Institute, Shrivenham, UK; and St Bartholomew's and The Royal London Hospitals, London, UK

5.1 Introduction and current state of the discipline

Until relatively recently radiological images were acquired using the same basic techniques of radiography and fluoroscopy that Röntgen himself employed. Whilst these basic techniques still form a major part of radiological investigation, they have been supplemented by newer techniques employing sophisticated computer technology, some of which rely on X-rays and others that employ radioactive materials, sound waves and magnetic fields. The majority of methods now employed permit images to be acquired and stored digitally.

The main medical radiological imaging techniques used for forensic examination of skeletonised or partially decomposed remains may be summarised as follows:

- Radiography: The term radiography is generally used to describe a static or 'still' image produced by means of a single exposure to X-rays (an energy form of ionising radiation). Such images are now usually recorded and stored digitally but were previously recorded photographically on X-ray film.

- Fluoroscopy: The term fluoroscopy is used to describe an image directly visualised in real-time motion produced by a continuous exposure to X-rays.

- Computed axial tomography: CAT or CT scanning employs a computerised X-ray machine that uses an array of photoreceptors to detect minute differences in attenuation of X-rays emitted by an X-ray tube as it rotates around the body or body part. A computer generates an image of the body part in the axial or cross-sectional plane and modern multidetector (MDCT) scanners permit multiplanar, multidirectional sectional images to be displayed and/or reconstructed as 3D images.

Forensic radiology of the deceased has, until very recently, been limited to the use of still-image radiography and occasionally fluoroscopy (Brogdon and Lichtenstein,

Forensic Ecology Handbook: From Crime Scene to Court, First Edition.
Edited by Nicholas Márquez-Grant and Julie Roberts.
© 2012 John Wiley & Sons, Ltd. Published 2012 by John Wiley & Sons, Ltd.

2011). Increasingly, however, some of the more complex imaging techniques, such as MDCT scanning, are being employed for post-mortem imaging.

5.2 Application of radiology to the analysis and identification of human remains*

Radiology is now widely used to assist in the analysis and identification of human remains, and the applications of the use of X-rays first suggested by Levinsohn, Angerer and Bordas comprise the main methods by which medical imaging contributes to the identification and investigative process (Brogdon and Lichtenstein, 2011; Goodman, 1995; Levinsohn, 1899). Radiological imaging has the advantage of enabling the examination of remains in a variety of states of decomposition from fully fleshed to completely skeletonised. As such, it affords the opportunity to obtain a considerable amount of data without the need to clean and completely deflesh the remains. It provides the investigative team with a rapid method of triage and classification by answering a number of fundamental questions:

1. **Establishing context**

   – Determination of human versus non-human remains.

   – Recognition of commingling.

   – Location and retrieval of artefacts and personal effects.

2. **Human identification**

   – Evaluation of the biological profile (age, sex, stature and ancestry).

   – Positive identification of individuals by comparison of ante-mortem and post-mortem radiological data.

3. **Analysis of injuries and retrieval of artifacts**

   – Interpretation of trauma.

   – Retrieval of forensic evidence.

5.2.1 Establishing context

5.2.1.1 *Human versus non-human*

In most cases involving animal bones, a simple visual examination is all that is necessary for the trained anatomist, osteologist or forensic anthropologist to determine

---

*Some material in the chapter has been reprinted with kind permission from Springer Science and Business Media: Bradley Adams and John Byrd (Eds.) Recovery Analysis and Identification of Commingled Human Remains, Chapter 8; The Use of Radiology in Mass Fatality Events, 2008, pp. 146–154, Mark Viner, © Humana Press.

non-human characteristics. In some cases, however, the most distinctive parts of the bones, the articular surfaces, may be missing due to fragmentation, decomposition or animal activity and, in such cases, radiographic examination of the bone structure and trabecular pattern can be useful to determine human from non-human remains (Brogdon 2011a; Chilvarquer *et al.*, 1987).

5.2.1.2 Recognition of commingling

In cases involving large amounts of fragmented remains, remains may be commingled and mixed with large amounts of debris and artefacts. Physical examination of such remains, particularly in cases of fire damage where there is a uniformity of discoloration of all samples retrieved, is both difficult and time-consuming. In such cases, radiological examination can prove useful both in determining the presence of one or more individuals but also in identifying and locating small body parts, especially teeth, which may otherwise be overlooked in the absence of a thorough and lengthy fingertip search (Goodman and Edelson, 2002; Kahana *et al.*, 1997; Viner, Cassidy and Treu, 1998).

5.2.1.3 Location and retrieval of artefacts and personal effects

In the same way, X-ray imaging can be utilised to detect and retrieve hazardous objects, personal effects, projectiles and other artefacts, and forensic evidence which have been retrieved together with the remains during body recovery or exhumation. This can be helpful especially when body fragmentation is extensive and has proved particularly useful in mass fatality incidents resulting from air disasters (Alexander and Foote, 1998; Mulligan *et al.*, 1988), explosions and terrorist incidents (Harcke, Bifano and Koeller 2002; Nye *et al.*, 1996) or where the body has been exhumed. In the latter case, it may also be useful to utilise X-ray techniques on-site to examine the associated debris excavated with the body in order to detect small items, such as jewellery or other personal effects that may have become disassociated from the body during decomposition (Gould, 2003; Tonello, 1998; Viner, 2008; Wessling and Loe, 2011) (Figure 5.1).

5.2.2 Human identification

5.2.2.1 Establishing the biological profile

Age estimation

The appearance and fusion of primary and secondary ossification centres within the developing skeleton follows a predetermined chronological pattern and, in the same way that a physical examination of the de-fleshed skeleton can determine age at the time of death, so can skeletal radiography deliver the same information in the case of less decomposed remains. There are a number of radiological standards

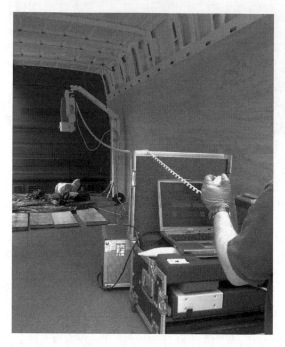

Figure 5.1   A portable direct digital X-ray system being used on-site to examine remains. In this particular case, the unit is located in the back of a van and is being powered by a small generator. Image by kind permission of Reveal Imaging Ltd.

for determination of bone age throughout the first two decades of life, based upon the appearance and fusion of the secondary ossification centres. The final epiphysis to fuse is the medial end of the clavicle, normally occurring during the mid to late twenties.

In addition to dental development, one of the most useful examinations in determining the age of children is radiography of the hand and wrist (e.g. Greulich and Pyle, 1959) (Figure 5.2), although examination of the knee, foot and ankle can also be helpful (Hansman, 1962; Hoerr, Pyle and Francis, 1962; Pyle and Hoerr, 1955; Scheuer and Black, 2004). In the mature skeleton, it is the degenerative changes that begin to appear primarily at the margins of the articular surfaces of major joints at around age 40 that will allow the experienced radiologist to estimate adult age within the range +/−5 to 10 years (Brogdon, 2011a). Calcification of the costal cartilages associated with the ribs and sternum may be readily visualised in people over 50, although it is sometimes observed in younger subjects (Mora *et al.*, 2001). Although chest radiography demonstrates this calcification, its specificity as an aging method is reduced due to similar amounts of mineralisation throughout adulthood (McCormick, 1980). It is, however, a quick, inexpensive method to obtain a general age estimate which can be used along with other anthropological examinations (e.g. pubic symphysis morphology). In the case of partially skeletonised remains,

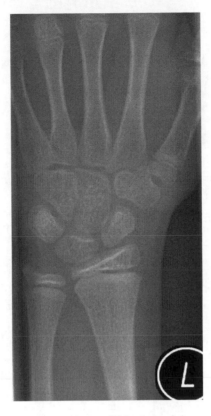

Figure 5.2 An X-ray of the wrist can be useful in determining age in sub-adult or juvenile individuals, as in this case of a child of around 11 years of age.

radiological examination using a multidetector CT scanner (MDCT) may be particularly useful for age estimation from the pubic symphysis (Dedouit *et al.*, 2011).

Sex estimation

Estimation of sex by skeletal radiology is unreliable until after puberty, as the features that distinguish male from female are not sufficiently developed until this point (Krogman and İşcan, 1986). Although on examination the appearance of the male skeleton is more substantial than the female, being generally heavier, more robust and the long bones of greater length, it is the examination of certain specific bones and their anatomical landmarks which is most useful in estimating the sex of an individual. In particular, the shape, size and geometry of the pelvis (Kurihara *et al.*, 1996; Rogers and Saunders, 1994; Sutherland and Suchey, 1991), the skull and mandible (Bass, 1986; Kurihara *et al.*, 1996), and the patterns of calcification of the costal (Navani, Shah and Levy, 1970), tracheobronchial, thyroid and arytenoid cartilages (Kurihara *et al.*, 1996) can be used to estimate sex from skeletal remains by radiological means (Brogdon, 2011a).

Stature estimation

Estimation of stature is often made by direct measurement from unfleshed human remains. The length of the femur is usually used, as this has been shown to be the most reliable bone (Trotter and Gleser, 1952, 1958). In the case of fleshed remains, the same measurements can be made radiographically, provided that correction for magnification is made. This can either be achieved by means of an adapted radiographic technique, applying a simple correction factor or by utilising modern imaging techniques, such as CT scanning and digital radiography.

CT scanners and digital X-ray systems can be calibrated to undertake this correction calculation automatically, thus allowing measurements to be made directly from the image. In the case of CT scanning, a scanogram is performed using the scanner to undertake an automated version of the manual process described above (Aitken *et al.*, 1985). Digital X-ray machines using a slit beam can also be used to take direct measurements, and many other direct digital X-ray machines can be calibrated to render accurate anatomical measurements from the resultant images (Beningfield *et al.*, 2003).

Estimation of ancestry

Determination of ancestry is challenging, especially when the remains are badly decomposed or skeletonised. Similar methods to those used by physical anthropologists to determine ancestry from skeletal remains can be applied radiographically with fleshed remains. In particular, examination of the skull and mandible (Bass, 1986; Fischman, 1985), the distal end of the femur (Craig, 1995) and the ratio of long-bone length can be useful in the estimation of population ancestry (Krogman and İşcan, 1986).

5.2.2.2 Positive identification of individuals by comparison of ante-mortem and post-mortem radiological data

In cases involving skeletonisation, fragmentation, decomposition, cremation, mutilation or other disfigurement, identification by means of the skeleton and highly resilient dentition assumes a greater importance and it is here that X-ray imaging comes into its own. Such incidents are often characterised by damage to the soft tissues caused by fire or water or severe disarticulation due to explosion or rapid deceleration injury.

Radiological identification of human remains requires specific and unique findings on post-mortem images to be matched exactly with ante-mortem images of the individual. In some cases, identification can be made from a series of relatively common or non-specific pathological anatomical changes that appear in identical locations in ante-mortem and post-mortem images. In other cases, a single unique feature is sufficient (Brogdon, 2011b). In 1927, Culbert and Law (Culbert and Law, 1927) made the first identification of human remains by comparison of ante-mortem and post-mortem radiographs of the frontal sinuses. The degree of human variation in sinus patterns, based on size, asymmetry, outline, partial sepia and supraorbital cells, makes effective comparison for identification possible (Kirk, Wood and Goldstein, 2002; Marlin, Clark and Standish, 1991; Nambiar, Naidu and Subramaniam, 1999).

Medical imaging has long been used for the identification of human remains and is well documented (Buchner, 1985; Craig, 1995; Jensen, 1991; Kahana and Hiss, 1997; Murphy, Spruill and Gantner, 1980; Sanders *et al.*, 1972; Schwartz and Woolridge, 1977). Radiology is used extensively in anthropological and odontological assessment of post-mortem and ante-mortem radiographs, records or other images for concordance as they represent an excellent source of data for comparison of anatomical features (Figure 5.3). Many specific cases have been reported in which radiology has played the leading role in the identification of human remains (Goodman and Edelson, 2002; Greulich and Pyle, 1959; Kahana *et al.*, 1997; Viner and Lichtenstein, 2011). Binda *et al.* (1999) even report on a case where radiology proved to be more accurate than DNA.

Radiographs taken for medical purposes are often required by statute to be retained for long periods of time. In the United Kingdom, for example, the

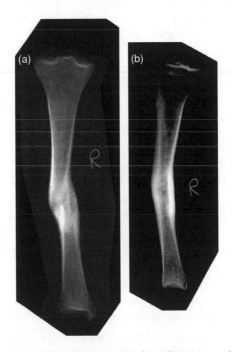

Figure 5.3   Healed fractures, such as this fracture of the tibia, can enable an identification to be made via comparison of ante-mortem and post-mortem images. Two projections of any fracture site, in the antero-posterior (a) and lateral (b) positions should be made during post-mortem examination. These are standard projections that are used in orthopaedic radiography to assess the healing fracture, and post-mortem films can thus be compared with any ante-mortem images that may be available.

Department of Health requires that radiographs are retained for eight years, and longer in the case of children (until the patient reaches their 25th year), and three years following death (Dimond, 2002). In many cases, particularly in privately run clinics, radiographs are routinely given to the patient for safe-keeping, and thus may be in existence for much longer than the statutory period. With the advent of digital imaging and the decreasing cost of digital storage, many institutions are retaining medical images far beyond their previously applied practice for X-ray film. Records are thus, on the whole, fairly accessible.

Despite the advent of more modern techniques, radiography still remains a widely used method accounting for well over half of the medical and dental X-ray examinations undertaken in the United Kingdom. Of these, the majority are X-rays of the teeth, chest and limb radiographs. This position echoes Brogdon's evaluation of the distribution of radiological examinations by body part and modality in the United States. As Brogdon asserts, examinations of the chest demonstrate consistency of bony structures over time, and extremities may contain useful radiographic identifiers due to previous injury, degenerative change or malformation. All of the above point to a wealth of useful ante-mortem data being available to the investigator, with the possibility of obtaining a clear and decisive identification if post-mortem and ante-mortem data can be matched (Brogdon, 2011b; Tanner *et al.*, 2000).

Radiographic examinations of the skull have declined dramatically since the advent of CT scanning, and ante-mortem radiographic data is thus less likely to be available. However, positive identification can be established by CT, either by comparison with other CT scans or some conventional radiographs (Brogdon, 2011b; Reichs and Dorion, 1992).

5.2.3   Analysis of injuries and retrieval of evidence

5.2.3.1   Interpretation of trauma

Radiology can be used to assist in determining the manner of death or the extent and mechanism of trauma. In cases of extensive trauma, individual demonstration of all fractures present after a fatal accident may be a time-consuming process and radiological examination simplifies the procedure. In addition, some fractures are difficult to demonstrate and are more adequately demonstrated using radiological methods, such as X-ray or CT scanning.

Radiological examination may yield far more than simply demonstrating the presence of fractures. It may be able to demonstrate the nature of the trauma that caused the fracture by determining the direction and impact of the force and, in some cases, may enable a fracture that has been caused by an assault to be differentiated from trauma sustained following an accidental fall (Figure 5.4) It is thus particularly useful in the investigation of suspected abuse of children and other vulnerable groups (Brogdon, 2011c; Brogdon and McDowell, 2011). MDCT scans and

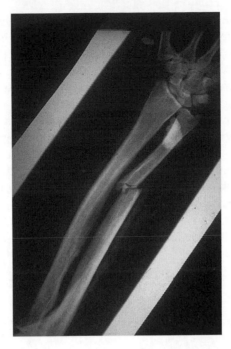

Figure 5.4 'Defence fracture' of the ulna caused by blunt force trauma to the forearm. Image by kind permission of the United Nations International Criminal Tribunal for the Former Yugoslavia.

surface scanning techniques may also allow three-dimensional modelling to identify directions of impact, and size and shape of weapons used to inflict trauma (Nather, Buck and Thali, 2011; Buck, Nather and Thali, 2011).

Radiology may also be of significance in proving the infliction of injury at various times by demonstrating healing and fresh (peri-mortem) fractures, and such evidence is essential to the concept of systematic abuse or torture (Brogdon, Vogel and McDowell, 2003). In some cases it may be particularly useful to identify sites of peri-mortem trauma which may be sampled for histological analysis.

The most obvious use of X-rays in cases of suspected homicide is to demonstrate bullets and other missiles within the body. Projectiles may be found at some considerable distance from the entry site and radiography can be used to locate these. The deployment of a dynamic imaging method, such as fluoroscopy, will accelerate the process of retrieving ballistic material (Di Maio, 1999; Brogdon and Messmer, 2011). This is particularly the case if the body is partially decomposed, has been subjected to fire or has been exhumed. In such cases, physical examination and location of ballistic material is often hindered by the uniform discolouration and can be a time-consuming process. Even if the missile is recovered without the aid of radiography, fragments of bullets or of bomb casings or contents can easily be missed in an unaided dissection and important information may be lost to the ballistics expert (Brogdon and Messmer, 2011; Tonello, 1998; Viner, 2008).

Other forms of homicide are also well illustrated by way of X-rays. Of significance is the radiography of the larynx in cases of strangulation, in which fractures of the thyroid cartilage or hyoid bone can be demonstrated, particularly if the cartilages are calcified, a process which increases with age. Radiology has proved particularly useful in assessing and documenting trauma in mass fatality incidents, resulting from air disasters (Alexander and Foote, 1998; Mulligan *et al.*, 1988; Viner and Lichtenstein, 2011), explosion and terrorist incidents including suicide attacks (Harcke *et al.*, 2002; Kahana *et al.*, 1997; Nye *et al.*, 1996; Society of Radiographers, 2005; Viner *et al.*, 2006). Radiological methods have also been employed extensively in the investigation of war crimes and human rights abuses involving the exhumation of buried human remains where radiology has assisted in the location of ballistic material, the evaluation of gunshot and/or explosive injuries and the investigation and documentation of any ante-mortem trauma (Gould, 2003; Tonello, 1998; Viner, 2001a, 2001b, 2008) (Figure 5.5).

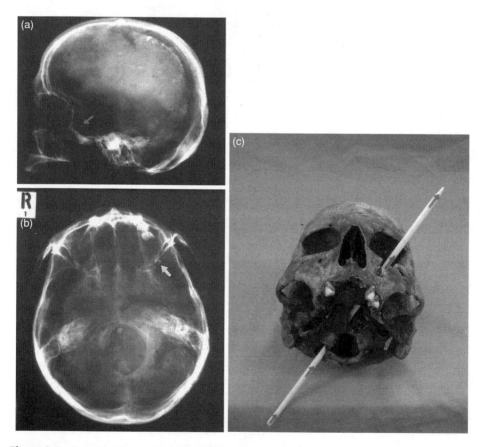

Figure 5.5 Lateral (a) and sub-mento-vertex (b) projections of the skull reveal ballistic traces within the skull in the area of the left orbit, confirming the path of a bullet from its entry site in the occipital bone to its exit through the left orbit (c). Images by kind permission of the United Nations International Criminal Tribunal for the Former Yugoslavia.

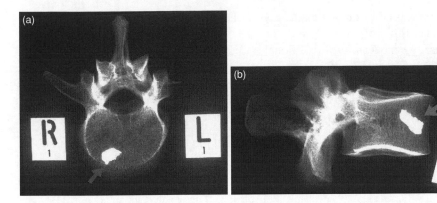

Figure 5.6 Initial X-ray examination of human remains revealed a ballistic fragment in the spine. This was further documented and localised by radiography of the lumbar vertebra prior to retrieval. Localisation is facilitated by two projections taken at 90 degrees; in this case supero-inferior (a) and lateral (b) projections. Images by kind permission of the United Nations International Criminal Tribunal for the Former Yugoslavia.

5.2.3.2   *Retrieval of forensic evidence*

As previously discussed, radiology is particularly useful in the location and retrieval of ballistic evidence related to gunshot wounds (Figure 5.6). Terrorist explosions are often caused by uniquely constructed home-made devices. Location and retrieval of fragments from the victims of the attack is often of vital forensic importance, and radiography is particularly indicated following such events. For this reason a full radiological survey is recommended in all such cases in order to locate all projectiles and fragments. Any radiographs that have been taken for the purpose of investigation can be retained as permanent records and, if necessary, used as exhibits at trial (Kahana *et al.*, 1997; Viner and Lichtenstein, 2011; Viner *et al.*, 2006). In such incidents, the systematic application of radiology has proved essential to the investigation and the identification of victims.

5.3   Conclusion

Radiology has a wide range of applications in the identification and analysis of human remains and associated artefacts and personal effects. It is an invaluable aid in the initial examination of suspected remains and related debris, enabling context to be established and facilitating the rapid identification and retrieval of small body parts, personal items and forensic evidence.

Its applications for human identification and analysis of trauma are especially valuable in situations involving partially decomposed remains or those which have been subjected to fire or fragmented by explosion. From assisting the determination of biological profile, through to determination of positive identification through comparison of ante-mortem and post-mortem images, radiology is an essential tool in the analysis of human remains and its application and deployment should be readily accessible.

Access to modern cross-sectional radiological techniques, such as MDCT scanning, for forensic and post-mortem investigation is steadily improving as the technology becomes both more economical and widely available. Greater levels of accuracy and the ability to examine subjects and display images in three dimensions offer an increasingly wide range of applications to the forensic investigator.

References

Aitken, A.G., Flodmark, O., Newman, D.E. *et al.* 1985. Leg length determination by CT digital radiography. *American Journal of Roentgenology* **144**: 613–615.

Alexander, C.J. and Foote, G.A. 1998. Radiology in forensic identification: the Mt Erebus disaster. *Australasian Radiology* **42**: 321–326.

Bass, W.M. 1986. Forensic anthropology. In M.F. Fierro and G.J. Loring (eds) *CAP Handbook for Postmortem Examination of Unidentified Remains; Developing Identification of Well Preserved, Decomposed, Burned, and Skeletonised Remains*. College of American Pathologists, Stokie, IL, pp. 85–110.

Beningfield, S., Potgieter, H., Nicol, A. *et al.* 2003. Report on a new type of trauma full-body digital X-ray machine. *Emergency Radiology* **10**: 23–29.

Binda, M., Cattaneo, C., Bogoni, A. *et al.* 1999. Identification of human skeletal remains: forensic radiology vs DNA. *La Radiologia Medica* (Torino) **97**: 409–411.

Brogdon, B.G. 2011a. Radiological identification: anthropological parameters. In M.J. Thali, M.D. Viner and B.G. Brogdon (eds) *Brogdon's Forensic Radiology*, 2nd edn. CRC Press, Boca Raton, FL, pp. 85–106.

Brogdon, B.G. 2011b. Radiological identification of individual remains. In M.J. Thali, M.D. Viner and B.G. Brogdon (eds) *Brogdon's Forensic Radiology*, 2nd edn. CRC Press, Boca Raton, FL, pp. 153–176.

Brogdon, B.G. 2011c. Child abuse. In M.J. Thali, M.D. Viner and B.G. Brogdon (eds) *Brogdon's Forensic Radiology*, 2nd edn. CRC Press, Boca Raton, FL, pp. 255–276.

Brogdon, B.G. and Lichtenstein, J.E. 2011. Forensic radiology in historical perspective. In M.J. Thali, M.D. Viner and B.G. Brogdon (eds) *Brogdon's Forensic Radiology*, 2nd edn. CRC Press, Boca Raton, FL, pp. 9–23.

Brogdon, B.G. and McDowell, J.D. 2011. Abuse of intimate partners and of the elderly. In M.J. Thali, M.D. Viner and B.G. Brogdon (eds) *Brogdon's Forensic Radiology*, 2nd edn. CRC Press, Boca Raton, FL, pp. 279–293.

Brogdon, B.G. and Messmer, M. 2011. Forensic radiology of gunshot wounds. In M.J. Thali, M.D. Viner and B.G. Brogdon (eds) *Brogdon's Forensic Radiology*, 2nd edn. CRC Press, Boca Raton, FL, pp. 211–240.

Brogdon, B.G., Vogel, H. and McDowell, J.D. 2003. *A Radiologic Atlas of Abuse, Torture, Terrorism, and Inflicted Trauma*. CRC Press, Boca Raton, FL.

Buchner, A. 1985. The identification of human remains. *International Dental Journal* **35**: 307–311.

Buck, U., Nather, S. and Thali, M.J. 2011. Using real 3D data for reconstruction. In M.J. Thali, M.D. Viner and B.G. Brogdon (eds) *Brogdon's Forensic Radiology*, 2nd edn. CRC Press, Boca Raton, FL, pp. 461–472.

Chilvarquer, I., Katz, J.O., Glassman, D.M. *et al.* 1987. Comparative radiographic study of human and animal long bone patterns. *Journal of Forensic Science* **32**: 1645–1654.

Craig, E.A. 1995. Intercondylar shelf angle: a new method to determine race from the distal femur. *Journal of Forensic Science* **40**: 777–782.

Culbert, W.L. and Law, F.M. 1927. Identification by comparison of roentgenograms of nasal accessory sinuses and mastoid processes. *The Journal of the American Medical Association* **88**: 1634–1636.

Dedouit F., Telmon, N., Rousseau, H. *et al.* 2011. Modern cross-sectional imaging in anthropology. In M.J. Thali, M.D. Viner and B.G. Brogdon (eds) *Brogdon's Forensic Radiology*, 2nd edn. CRC Press, Boca Raton, FL, pp. 107–126.

Dimond, B. 2002. *Legal Aspects of Radiography and Radiology*. Blackwell Publishing, Oxford.

Di Maio, V.J.M. 1999. *Gunshot Wounds: Practical Aspects of Firearms, Ballistics and Forensic Techniques*, 2nd edn. CRC Press, Boca Raton, FL.

Fischman, S.L. 1985. The use of medical and dental radiographs in identification. *International Dental Journal* **35**: 301–306.

Goodman, N.R. and Edelson, L.B. 2002. The efficiency of an X-ray screening system at a mass disaster. *Journal of Forensic Science* **47**: 127–130.

Goodman, P.C. 1995. The new light: discovery and introduction of the X-ray. *American Journal of Roentgenology* **165**: 1041–1045.

Gould, P. 2003. X-ray detectives turn images into evidence. *Diagnostic Imaging* (Special Edition).

Greulich, W.W. and Pyle, S.I. 1959. *Radiographic Atlas of Skeletal Development of the Hand and Wrist*. Stanford University Press, Stanford.

Hansman, C.F. 1962. Appearance and fusion of ossification centers in the human skeleton. *Americal Journal of Roentgenology* **88**: 476–482.

Harcke, H.T., Bifano, J.A. and Koeller, K.K. 2002. Forensic radiology: response to the Pentagon Attack on September 11, 2001. *Radiology* **223**: 7–8.

Hoerr, N.L., Pyle, S.I. and Francis, C.C. 1962. *Radiological Atlas of the Foot and Ankle*. Charles C Thomas, Springfield, IL.

Jensen, S. 1991. Identification of human remains lacking skull and teeth. A case report with some methodological considerations. *American Journal of Forensic Medicine & Pathology* **12**: 93–97.

Kahana, T. and Hiss, J. 1997. Identification of human remains: forensic radiology. *Journal of Clinical Forensic Medicine* **4**: 7–15.

Kahana, T., Ravioli, J.A., Urroz, C.L. and Hiss, J. 1997. Radiographic identification of fragmentary human remains from a mass disaster. *American Journal of Forensic Medicine & Pathology* **18**: 40–44.

Kirk, N.J., Wood, R.E. and Goldstein, M. 2002. Skeletal identification using the frontal sinus region: a retrospective study of 39 cases. *Journal of Forensic Science* **47**: 318–323.

Krogman, W.M. and İşcan, M.Y. 1986 *The Human Skeleton in Forensic Medicine*, 2nd edn. Charles C Thomas, Springfield, IL.

Kurihara, Y., Kurihara, Y., Ohashi, K. *et al.* 1996. Radiologic evidence of sex differences: is the patient a woman or a man? *American Journal of Roentgenology* **167**: 1037–1040.

Levinsohn. 1899. Beiträge zur Feststellung der Identität. *Arch Kriminal – Anthrop Kriminalistik* **2**: 211–220.

McCormick, W.F. 1980. Mineralization of the costal cartilages as an indicator of age: preliminary observations. *Journal of Forensic Science* **25**: 736–741.

Marlin, D.C., Clark, M.A. and Standish, S.M. 1991. Identification of human remains by comparison of frontal sinus radiographs: a series of four cases. *Journal of Forensic Science* **36**: 1765–1772.

Mora, S., Boechat, M.I., Pietka, E. *et al.* 2001. Skeletal age determination of children of European and African descent: applicability of the Greulich and Pyle standards. *Pediatric Research* **50**: 624–628.

Mulligan, M.E., McCarthy, M.J., Wippold, F.J. *et al.* 1988. Radiologic evaluation of mass casualty victims: lessons from the Gander, Newfoundland, accident. *Radiology* **168**: 229–233.

Murphy, W.A., Spruill, F.G. and Gantner, G.E. 1980. Radiologic identification of unknown human remains. *Journal of Forensic Science* **25**: 727–735.

Nambiar, P., Naidu, M.D. and Subramaniam, K. 1999. Anatomical variability of the frontal sinuses and their application in forensic identification. *Clinical Anatomy* **12**: 16–19.

Nather, S., Buck, U. and Thali, M.J. 2011. Photogrametry based optical scanning. In M.J. Thali, M.D. Viner and B.G. Brogdon (eds) *Brogdon's Forensic Radiology*, 2nd edn. CRC Press, Boca Raton, FL, pp. 365–388.

Navani, S., Shah, J.R. and Levy, P.S. 1970. Determination of sex by costal cartilage calcification. *American Journal of Roentgenology* **108**: 771–774.

Nye, P.J., Tytle, T.L., Jarman, R.N. and Eaton, B.G. 1996. The role of radiology in the Oklahoma City bombing. *Radiology* **200**: 541–543.

Pyle, S.I. and Hoerr, N.L. 1955. *Atlas of Skeletal Development of the Knee*. Charles C Thomas, Springfield, IL.

Reichs, K. and Dorion, R.B.J. 1992. The use of computed tomography (CT) scans in the analysis of frontal sinus configuration. *Canadian Society of Forensic Science Journal* **25**: 1–16.

Rogers, T. and Saunders, S. 1994. Accuracy of sex determination using morphological traits of the human pelvis. *Journal of Forensic Science* **39**: 1047–1056.

Sanders, I., Woesner, M.E., Ferguson, R.A. and Noguchi, T.T. 1972. A new application of forensic radiology: identification of deceased from a single clavicle. *American Journal of Roentgenology* **115**: 619–622.

Scheuer, L. and Black, S. 2004. *The Juvenile Skeleton*. Academic Press, London.

Schwartz, S. and Woolridge, E.D. 1977. The use of panoramic radiographs for comparisons in cases of identification. *Journal of Forensic Science* **22**: 145–146.

Society of Radiographers. 2005. Radiographers help identify London Bombing victims. *Synergy*, September Issue: 1.

Sutherland, L.D. and Suchey, J.M. 1991. Use of the ventral arc in pubic sex determination. *Journal of Forensic Science* **36**: 501–511.

Tanner, R.J., Wall, B.F., Shrimpton, P.C. *et al.* 2000. *Frequency of Medical and Dental X-ray Examinations in the UK, 1997–98*. National Radiological Protection Board, UK.

Tonello, B. 1998. Mass grave investigations. *Paper presented at the Imaging Science & Oncology*, British Institute of Radiology.

Trotter, M. and Gleser, G.C. 1952. Estimation of stature from long bones of American Whites and Negroes. *American Journal of Physical Anthropology* **10**: 463–514.

Trotter, M. and Gleser, G.C. 1958. A re-evaluation of estimation of stature based on measurements of stature taken during life and of long bones after death. *American Journal of Physical Anthropology* **16**: 79–123.

Viner, M.D. 2001a. Forensic investigation: the role of radiography. *European Radiology* **11**(Suppl.): 95.

Viner, M.D. 2001b. The radiographers role in forensic investigation. *Hold Putsen: Journal of the Norwegian Society of Radiographers*, 9/2001, October, Oslo.

Viner, M.D. 2008. The use of radiology in mass fatality incidents. In B. Adams and J. Byrd (eds) *Recovery, Analysis and Identification of Co-mingled Human Remains*. Humana Press, Totowa, NJ, pp. 145–179.

Viner, M.D and Lichtenstein, J.E. 2011. Radiology in mass casualty situations. In M.J. Thali, M.D. Viner and B.G. Brogdon (eds) *Brogdon's Forensic Radiology*, 2nd edn. CRC Press, Boca Raton, FL, pp. 177–198.

Viner, M.D., Cassidy, M. and Treu, V. 1998. The role of radiography in a disaster investigation. Paper presented at the Imaging Science and Oncology, British Institute of Radiology.

Viner, M.D., Rock, C., Hunt, N. *et al.* 2006. Forensic radiography: Response to the London suicide bombings on 7th July 2005. Paper presented at the American Academy of Forensic Sciences 58th Scientific Meeting, Seattle, WA.

Wessling, R. and Loe, L. 2011. The Fromelles Project: Organizational and operational structures of a large-scale mass grave excavation and on-site anthropological analysis. Paper presented at the American Academy of Forensic Sciences 63rd Scientific Meeting, Chicago, IL.

6

DNA analysis for victim identification

Michael Walbank and Andrew McDonald
Cellmark Forensic Services, Abingdon, UK

6.1   Introduction

DNA in forensics has been used since the discovery in 1984 of DNA fingerprints by Sir Alec Jeffreys (Jeffreys, Wilson and Thein, 1985), who also produced the first DNA profile in 1987. The identification of semi-decomposed or skeletonised remains whether an individual case or hundreds of individuals in mass fatalities, relies on a number of techniques including forensic anthropology, forensic odontology and other physical features. DNA has nevertheless been used as a primary means of identification of victims and in England and Wales, many coroners (and their equivalent in other countries), will wait to confirm identity after DNA analysis, even though forensic odontology may have provided a positive identification. It is part of the role of the Forensic Pathologist and at times the Forensic Anthropologist to sample tissue for DNA analysis. This chapter will cover the taking of tissue samples from deceased individuals and unidentified body parts for DNA analysis along with the collection of appropriate reference samples. In addition we will also discuss DNA profiling in the context of victim identification. DNA applications in forensics as well as background information on the history and development of the field can be found elsewhere (Buckleton, Triggs and Walsh, 2005; Butler, 2005).

6.2   Taking DNA samples from the deceased

Cadavers may be entirely intact or hugely fragmented and the state of decomposition may be relatively little or very advanced, depending on a number of factors. The state of decomposition of the body has a big effect on determining the DNA protocol required. If a body is largely intact and it shows little decomposition, then sampling is straightforward. If a body is rapidly decomposing, or in an advanced

Forensic Ecology Handbook: From Crime Scene to Court, First Edition.
Edited by Nicholas Márquez-Grant and Julie Roberts.
© 2012 John Wiley & Sons, Ltd. Published 2012 by John Wiley & Sons, Ltd.

state of decomposition, then the choice of which samples to take for DNA identifications becomes more critical as the DNA in the soft, fleshy parts of the body may have deteriorated to such an extent that the ability to obtain complete STR (short tandem repeat) profiles (see below) from the victims becomes significantly reduced.

Prior to sampling in the mortuary, the necessary equipment is recommended:

- Face masks.

- Disposable gloves (e.g. latex or nitrile).

- Disposable scalpels (sterile and individually packaged) (e.g. Swann-Morton 10A).

- Disposable plastic forceps (sterile and individually packaged).

- Range of sterile, plastic containers (mostly 7 ml and 30 ml volumes, but also some 60 ml and 120 ml volumes).

- Disposable white suits (e.g. Tyvek suits) or scrubs.

During a post-mortem examination, there may be many people around the examination table, each of whom has their own responsibility (e.g. pathologist, mortuary technicians, scribes and photographers). Although best practice would dictate that all individuals around the body need to wear hairnets and face masks and are also double-gloved, the reality may be quite different. All individuals should, at the very least, be wearing disposable (e.g. latex or nitrile) gloves (and ideally one pair of gloves over another pair of gloves), but whether it is really necessary to be wearing face masks and hairnets is debatable. The reason for this debate is that, as much as possible, any sample being collected for DVI (disaster victim identification) DNA purposes should be taken from a protected area of the body part (i.e. from an area that is only exposed during the post-mortem examination). When it comes to the point in the post-mortem examination where a suitable sample for DNA analysis is being considered, then all involved in the examination should be aware of the risks of them contaminating any sample and, if possible, step back from the table so only those involved in the searching for and taking of the DNA sample are around the body part at that time.

Based on our own experience, we would recommend that when considering which body part to sample for the identification of the deceased, it is best to avoid, if at all possible, areas that show exposed injuries (e.g. muscle tissue around an open wound). Such areas may have tissue or blood from other injured individuals present on them such that any DNA analysis runs the risk of generating mixed DNA profiles. Instead, in order to avoid unnecessary further trauma to the body, it is worth considering looking for suitable samples at a wound site but taken from deeper within the body where there is no risk of impaction of some other individual's DNA.

Fresh muscle tissue is bright pink in colour but as decomposition advances, the pink colouration of the tissue becomes brown. In a burnt body, initial observations may be misleading as charring of the body may result in the blackening of the body part but by asking for the pathologist to cut into the body part, pink muscle may become apparent. It may be necessary to ask the pathologist to cut into various areas of the body part to look for some pink-coloured muscle. If any bright pink-coloured muscle tissue is observed, then this should be sampled for DNA analysis.

Depending on the state of decomposition, there may be a need to cut into brown-coloured muscle tissue to seek out some slightly pink-coloured material. If there is no bright pink-coloured muscle tissue available, any slightly pink-coloured muscle tissue that is observed should be sampled for DNA analysis.

When suitable muscle tissue is exposed, it will then be necessary for the pathologist to use a new, sterile, pre-packed disposable scalpel, as well as a new set of disposable forceps, if required, to section the sample for DNA analysis from the body part. The DNA expert may be required to remind the pathologist that new, disposable scalpel and forceps need to be used as the pathologist may not be aware of issues about DNA cross-contamination. A small piece of tissue sample (approximately 5 mm × 5 mm × 5 mm for pink-coloured tissue or a larger piece (no more than 2 cm^3) of tissue showing signs of advanced decomposition should be collected into a labelled plastic container (e.g. specimen pot or universal).

If no pink-coloured muscle tissue is available, it will then become necessary to consider other sample types. In terms of ease of analysis, the next sample type to be considered would be bone marrow (particularly from the rib or sternum). Bone marrow from the rib or sternum, when fresh, is very soft and waxy and a small section of approximately 2–3 cm in length should be sampled from these (possibly requiring the use of rib shears), and collected into a labelled plastic container (e.g. specimen pot or universal). If possible to do so, it may be necessary to inform the pathologist or mortuary technician that the rib shears will need to be rinsed thoroughly before being used again. The potential for cross-contamination of samples must be borne in mind when advising about sample collection for DNA analysis.

If no pink-coloured muscle tissue, rib or sternum is available, it may become necessary to collect a tooth or to sample another type of bone for analysis. This involves the most time-consuming laboratory procedures and should only be considered when no other sample, likely to yield a DNA profile, is available. Keeping the size of the sample being collected to a relatively small piece (i.e. approximately 2 cm^3) can assist with reducing the amount of preparation work required at the laboratory before DNA analysis can be undertaken. In order of preference, any tooth (as long as there is no obvious signs of decay or other disease and no obvious signs of dental work such as a filling) should be removed from the jaw. Alternatively, if sampling a tooth is not possible, a relatively small piece of any bone could be taken. Many different types of bone sample (e.g. skull bone, femur, innominate, metatarsal, radius, ulna) have been analysed at the laboratory and all appear to be good sources of DNA. The tooth or bone sample should be collected into a labelled plastic container (e.g. specimen pot or universal). If bone-cutting equipment is used it may also be necessary to inform the pathologist or mortuary technician that the equipment will need to be rinsed thoroughly before being used again. As before, the potential for cross-contamination of samples must be borne in mind when advising about sample collection for DNA analysis.

It may be that the body part being examined has no muscle tissue or bone associated with it. Examples of body parts falling into this category would include body organs (e.g. spleen, kidney, lung, brain). All of these can be sampled for DNA analysis but it may be necessary for the DNA expert to liaise with the pathologist in order to find an area of the organ that appears either undamaged or shows the least decomposition. It is difficult to describe here what to look for specifically but by discussing the need for some part of the organ that shows the least deterioration with the pathologist, a suitable area will then be decided upon and sampled as for muscle tissue (i.e. new disposable scalpel and new forceps, if required). As for muscle tissue, if the sample appears to show very little in the way of decomposition then only a small piece of the organ would be required (approximately $5 \, \text{mm}^3$) but if decomposition is apparent then a larger piece would be needed (no more than $2 \, \text{cm}^3$). The sampled piece of body organ should be collected into a labelled plastic container (e.g. specimen pot or universal).

Some samples, such as body fat, have very little realistic prospect of generating a DNA profile and therefore there is little point in sampling them for DNA. Hairs, liquid blood and mouth swabs should also be avoided, if possible, and should only be considered if there is no muscle, tooth or bone to analyse. Table 6.1 provides a ranking recommended by the authors, in their own experience of deceased and body parts from mass fatality incidents or DVI.

6.2.1   Reconciliation of body parts to specific individuals

As with the identification of the deceased, the state of the body parts has a big effect on the sampling procedure. Also, before any sampling is carried out, a decision is required as to which body parts to sample. In some cases, size criteria is established where body parts below a certain size are deemed to be too small to require DNA analysis. For example, following terrorist incidents in London in 2005, the Coroner made the decision that only body parts that had a volume of greater than $125 \, \text{cm}^3$ (i.e. would be too big to fit into a container $5 \, \text{cm} \times 5 \, \text{cm} \times 5 \, \text{cm}$ in size) would be considered for DNA analysis. Exceptions were made for smaller parts that were clearly identifiable (e.g. tips of fingers and fragments of ear or body organs such as pieces of brain and kidney and identifiable bone fragments) by the forensic anthropologists. For body parts that fell into this category, if there was some material present that might yield a DNA profile, then this was sampled in order to establish the identity of the individual from whom the smaller pieces of body parts originated.

6.2.2   Storage of DNA samples

After a section of tissue or bone has been obtained from the body or body part, the collected sample will be passed to the person responsible for exhibiting the item (usually by a designated Police Exhibit Officer). This will involve generating a

Table 6.1 A guide, in order of preference, for deciding which samples to take in a DVI incident.

Item type	Sample	Comments
1. Bright pink muscle tissue	Muscle tissue showing little sign of decomposition. Approx. 5 mm × 5 mm × 5 mm sample required.	May be necessary to cut into various areas of the body part to seek out fresh, pink-coloured muscle tissue.
2. Pale pink muscle tissue	Muscle tissue showing signs of decomposition. Avoid sampling areas of brown-coloured muscle or charred muscle (in burnt remains). A larger piece of muscle tissue may need to be sampled depending on the state of decomposition. No more than 2 cm × 2 cm × 2 cm would be required.	May be necessary to cut into various areas of the body part to seek out any pink-coloured muscle tissue. Once the body or body part has been extensively tested, choose the most pink-coloured muscle for sampling.
3. Body organs	When no muscle tissue sample is available, it is worth considering any body organ sample. Treat sampling as for muscle tissue (approx. 5 mm × 5 mm × 5 mm for fresh material but a larger amount for material showing signs of decomposition – no more than 2 cm × 2 cm × 2 cm would be required).	May need to liaise closely with the pathologist to recognise areas of body organs showing least signs of damage or decomposition. Can be difficult to assess but it may be necessary to sample bone if body organ appears 'cooked'. Still sample 'cooked' body organ tissue if no other sample available.
4. Rib marrow	Ribs showing little sign of decomposition have a soft, waxy marrow. Sample a small section of the rib (approx. 2–3 cm in length) containing the soft marrow.	Avoid any damaged ends of the rib and investigate an area of the ribs or sternum that appears less damaged or decomposed.
5. Tooth	For tooth samples, any tooth can be taken for sampling but it must not contain a cap, crown or filling and should not show signs of disease.	Tooth should be removed from jaw, if possible. If only tooth with filling is available, then it will necessary to discuss the removal of the filling by a forensic odontologist prior to the tooth being submitted for DNA analysis.
6. Bone	Wide range of bone samples is good for DNA analysis. Only sample if there is no other sample available that is likely to yield a DNA profile. Can be protected when rest of body part shows extensive charring. Sample a small section of bone (approx. 2 cm × 2 cm × 2 cm in size).	Try to avoid any damaged bone, if possible. Keeping the sampled piece to a small size can assist with the laboratory analysis procedure.

unique item number for the sample and recording on an exhibit list the exact details of the sample against the unique item number. The sample may then be packaged into a tamper evident bag, the details of the sample and its continuity written onto the bag and then the item put to one side for DNA analysis or put elsewhere for those not requiring DNA analysis.

Ideally the samples requiring DNA analysis should be placed into a freezer (approximately $-20°C$ or colder) as soon as possible to prevent further decomposition. Realistically, especially in an incident in a location where facilities are limited, this may not be possible and anything that can be done to slow down the decomposition process should be considered. For example there may not be sufficient freezers for the samples so attempts should be made to keep the samples as cool as possible until they can be transported to a freezer. This may mean putting the samples into a refrigerator ($+4°C$) or cool boxes with ice packs inside or, at the very least, keeping the samples out of the sun and in the coolest available place. If freezers are not available, it may be necessary for the DNA expert to inform the person in authority how important it is to get the DNA samples into a freezer as quickly as possible to prevent further decomposition, since decomposition will reduce the ability to obtain a DNA profile from the sample.

6.3   Collection of reference samples for victim identification

In order for deceased individuals to be identified, or body parts attributed to individuals, it is necessary to have appropriate reference samples from which DNA profiles can be obtained for comparison with the DNA profiles obtained from unidentified individuals or body parts. These reference samples can be taken from individuals themselves (direct or surrogate reference samples) or from blood relatives.

6.3.1   Direct reference samples

Where there is clear provenance as to the origin of a sample, samples taken directly from identified individuals can be used for identification purposes. Examples of these are medical samples, samples taken from identified individuals who may be missing body parts (e.g. in an explosion), UK DNA database samples.

6.3.2   Surrogate reference samples

Where no direct reference sample is available, personal effects can be used to generate DNA profiles for missing or unidentified individuals (Table 6.2). These should ideally take the form of personal items unlikely to have been used by others, such as toothbrushes and razors, which only the individual in question will have had

Table 6.2 Recommended surrogate samples.

DNA sources	Commonly available	Might be available

Good sources of DNA	Toothbrushes
	Razors
		Blood cards from PKU newborn
		  screening
		Pathology specimens/paternity
		  samples
		Reference samples from military
		  personnel

Fair sources of DNA	Hairbrushes and combs Clothing Used cups and drinking glasses Cigarette ends	Histology slides (e.g. cervical smears) Fingernail clippings Mouth guards
Poor sources of DNA	Jewellery Watches	Dentures

intimate contact with. If items of this nature are not available then jewellery, clothing or footwear can be considered but there is a greater chance of these items having DNA present on them from other parties causing interpretational difficulties in assigning a profile to the owner.

6.3.3   Next of kin samples

Where no direct or surrogate reference sample is available, individuals can be identified by comparison to DNA profiles obtained from their relatives. These should be from closely related biological relatives and ideally parents, children or full siblings. Samples from more distant relatives can be used but the results may not be as conclusive. There are a number of ways to taking these samples but the most common is to swab for cells from the mouth (Butler, 2005).

6.4   DNA laboratory analysis

In order to develop an understanding of DNA laboratory analysis and the role it plays in victim identification, it is first necessary to consider the structure and function of DNA itself.

6.4.1   DNA structure and function

DNA is a complex molecule found inside almost all cell types within the human body (the exception being red blood cells) and carries an individual's genetic blueprint. An individuals' DNA is separated into distinct paired molecules called chromosomes and in humans there are 23 pairs or 46 chromosomes in total.

Each chromosome is comprised of a long double-stranded molecule made up of a long chain consisting of four basic complementary repeating units called bases: adenosine, thymine, guanine and cytosine. It is the order of these bases along each chromosome that carries an individuals' genetic code (e.g. see Butler, 2005).

An individuals DNA is inherited from their biological parents with half coming from each parent. As a result closely related individuals will tend to have more of their DNA in common than unrelated individuals.

As the DNA that an individual inherits from its parents is random siblings can share greatly varied amounts of DNA. Conversely, as genetic relationships between individuals become more distant then the amount of DNA they have common also decreases.

6.4.2 DNA in forensics

Although humans share a very high percentage of their DNA with each other there are a small percentage of regions that show wide degrees of variability between individuals and it is these so-called hyper-variable regions (known as short tandem repeats or STRs) – that enable DNA to be used as a means of identifying or discriminating between individuals.

STRs do not carry any genetic coding information as such and are regarded as 'spacer' DNA, acting to separate the coding regions. They are made up of short sequences of only a few base pairs in length which are then repeated several times. It is the number of these repeat units that vary from individual to individual. Such STR regions are found throughout the human genome and when a number of these are used in combination with each other they provide a very powerful means for individualisation.

6.4.2.1 The DNA profiling process

When a sample has been submitted by a police force to the laboratory and the correct forms have been filled with regard to continuity of the item (submission form, receipt form, etc.) and other administrative protocols have been undertaken, sample processing takes place, involving a series of distinct laboratory procedures: extraction, quantification, amplification and electrophoresis.

- *Extraction:* The sample, or a small piece of it, is incubated with reagents (buffers and enzymes) designed to break down any cellular material present thereby releasing any DNA contained. DNA extraction procedures vary depending on the type of sample in question, the amount of DNA it may contain and the physical nature of the sample itself. Good sources of DNA such as mouth swabs, blood and fresh tissue samples require relatively straightforward procedures, whereas items such as bones or teeth, where the cellular material is tightly bound into the structure of the material, require more rigorous and lengthy procedures to extract the DNA they contain. Bone will require decontamination, sectioning, grinding,

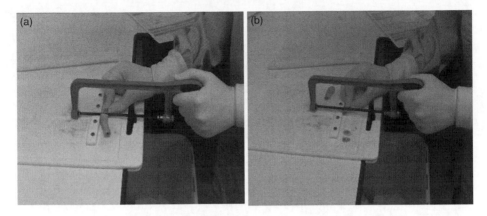

Figure 6.1 The bones are sampled (e.g. section of midshaft of a long bone) according to condition and quality. Images courtesy of Cellmark Forensic Services.

digesting and purifying (Figures 6.1, 6.2 and 6.3). In addition, old items or items that have been subjected to harmful environmental conditions may also require more specialist extraction procedures in order to maximise the DNA recovered. These procedures should be undertaken in optimum lab conditions to avoid contamination especially in the extraction process where general requirements tend to be, in our experience, the use of lab shoes or shoe overalls, followed by putting on a face mask and hairnet, after which a clean suit (e.g. Tyvek suit) is put on. Lastly disposable sterile gloves will be put on (two gloves on each hand).

- *Quantification:* In order to optimise the subsequent amplification stage it is important to establish the concentration of the DNA extracted from any given sample. This is done by precisely measuring with a Real-Time PCR system, the concentration of DNA in a small amount of the extract. Typically DNA

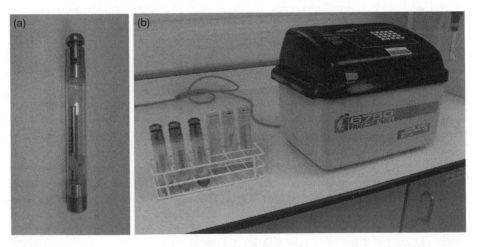

Figure 6.2 The bone sections are placed into a polycarbonate cylinder along with a magnetic crushing rod used for pulverisation. Images courtesy of Cellmark Forensic Services.

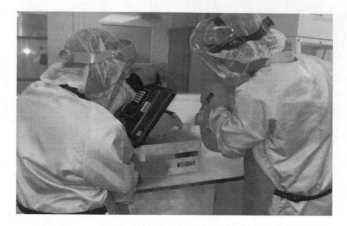

Figure 6.3 The samples in the polycarbonate cylinders are frozen using liquid nitrogen and then crushed into a fine powder. Image courtesy of Cellmark Forensic Services.

concentrations vary from 0.00 nanograms (ng) to over 100 ng per microlitre (μl) of extract (1 ng = 1 billionth of a gram, 1 μl = 1 thousandth of a millilitre) with the amplification process being optimised for 1 ng/μl of DNA.

- *Amplification:* A cyclical chemical reaction called the polymerase chain reaction (PCR) is used to copy the DNA sites being tested many times over in order to bring them to a detectable level. A standard PCR reaction typically uses 28 cycles thereby achieving an amplification rate of 2×10^{28} equating to each DNA site being copied over 200 million times.

- *Electrophoresis:* The DNA sites within each sample amplified during the PCR reaction, need to be visualised so that profiling data can be attached to them and a DNA profile determined for the sample itself. This is achieved by running a small amount of the PCR product derived from a sample through an electro-conductive gel which allows the DNA pieces to be separated according to their size – small pieces migrating through the gel faster than big pieces. As each piece of DNA reaches the end of the gel it passes a detector which records its size. Computer software converts this sizing data into the profiling results for each of the DNA sites tested so allowing an STR profile to be generated for each sample.

6.5 Common DNA profiling tests

In the United Kingdom there are a number of DNA profiling tests that are commonly employed in forensic casework:

- **SGM:** The test was originally used for supplying profiles to the UK National DNA Database from 1995 to 2001. It tested six DNA STR regions and a sex-determining marker and had a discriminating power of approximately 1 in 50 million.

- **SGM+:** Introduced in the United Kingdom in 2001, SGM+ was the successor to SGM. It includes the six STR regions and the sex marker from SGM with the addition of four further STR regions designed to give it greater discriminating power (1 in 1 billion) than SGM whilst remaining compatible with previous SGM samples.

- **Identifiler:** This test includes the 10 STRs and the sex marker used in SGM+ with the addition of a further five loci which allow greater discrimination between closely related individuals. Consequently it is extensively used in paternity testing and in the identification of unidentified deceased individuals when reference samples are to be submitted from close family members.

- **Powerplex16:** This test includes 13 of the STRs and the sex marker present in Identifiler with the addition of two alternative STRs known to be highly variable between individuals. Consequently it is of use when the further investigation of close family relationships is required.

- **Y-STRs:** This test uses STR regions located only on the male Y-chromosome. As females have no Y-chromosome Y-STRs can only be passed on through the male line of a family, hence all male members of the same family line will have the same Y-chromosome and consequently the same Y-STR profile. This test is therefore used to investigate familial relationships where males are thought to be related. This is particularly useful when the relatives in question are not biologically close (e.g. grandfather and grandchild). In the United Kingdom there are no Y-STR databases available so profiles from unidentified individuals cannot be searched as a means of establishing identity.

- **Mitochondrial DNA:** Mitochondria are small organs ('organelles') responsible for cellular respiration. They have their own DNA and are present in all cells in large numbers. Mitochondria are inherited maternally; hence all maternally related individuals will have the same mitochondrial profile. This test is therefore used to investigate relationships where individuals are thought to be maternally inherited. In addition, because there are many mitochondria in every cell, mitochondrial profiles can be obtained from degraded samples where nuclear STR DNA testing has failed to produce a profile, but there must either be direct reference samples available from the individuals in question or reference samples from confirmed maternal relatives in order for comparisons to be made. As with Y-STRs there are no mitochondrial DNA databases available in the United Kingdom at present so profiles from unidentified individuals cannot be searched as a means of establishing identity.

6.5.1 High-sensitivity DNA profiling tests

Under certain circumstances, samples may unsuitable for profiling with standard DNA profiling techniques. This occurs in cases where either the age of the sample has lead to the degradation of the DNA or where the nature of an incident has caused? DNA degradation such as in the case of bodies exposed to fires or chemicals.

In these circumstances there are further DNA profiling tests that may still yield DNA profiles. These tests are more sensitive than conventional profiling tests and are therefore able to detect lower quantities of DNA. However, this increased sensitivity also makes these tests more prone to detecting additional spurious DNA components present in a sample, introduced either during the incident itself (impaction and commingling of remains), during collection at the scene or during the subsequent examination and processing of the sample in the laboratory. The presence of this additional DNA can make the subsequent interpretation of the results obtained by these methods difficult.

The different techniques (see also Buckleton *et al.*, 2005; Butler, 2005) that can be employed are:

- **Increased Amplification Cycle Number:** Additional amplification cycles (see below) which are typically 30 or 34 instead of 28 are used to increase the effective sensitivity of standard DNA profiling processes.

- **Enhancement:** The post-amplification products of standard DNA profiling tests are concentrated and artefacts (unused reagents) from the amplification process are removed to increase the detection sensitivity of the electrophoresis process.

- **Minifiler:** Minifiler is a specialist DNA profiling test in itself which has been designed for use on samples containing degraded or low-levels of DNA.

6.5.2   Profiling results and the matching process

DNA profiling results appear as a series of peaks representing the combination of STR components comprising the DNA profile of each sample. This DNA profile can then be compared to DNA profiles obtained from other relevant samples submitted from the same case. These may be reference samples from known individuals, tissue samples from unidentified individuals/body parts or reference samples from family members.

6.5.2.1   Match probabilities

For two DNA profiles to be considered to be a match and therefore for the two samples from which the profiles have arisen be considered to have originated from the same source, all the components represented in each profile must match each other exactly. If all of the components do not match each other then the profiles themselves are considered to be non-matching; it would therefore be concluded that they cannot have arisen from the same source.

For fully matching profiles it is then possible to carry out a statistical evaluation of this match in terms of the probability of obtaining the match if the two profiles originated from different and unrelated individuals and the match had arisen by chance. This calculation is known as a 'match probability' and is based on the respective frequency with which each component in the profile occurs in the population at large. These frequencies are combined to give the overall match probability for the given profile.

Typically in the United Kingdom, for matches between two SGM+ or Identifiler profiles this probability would be reported as being approximately 1 in 1 billion and would be accompanied by a verbal assessment of the strength of the match in terms of the support it provides for the proposed identification or match. This wording is taken from a pre-determined scale: no support, weak support, moderate, strong, very strong, or extremely strong support.

6.5.2.2 *Next of kin samples and likelihood ratios*

For instances where the profile from a sample of unknown origin is being compared to a reference profile of a relative of a missing person there would not be an expectation of obtaining completely matching profiles and consequently more complex statistical calculations are required. This is done by calculating the probability of them sharing DNA components as a result of the proposed relationship versus the probability of them sharing components by chance if they are unrelated. The results of these analyses are expressed as a ratio of these two probabilities, this is known as a likelihood ratio (LR).

6.5.3 Databases

If there are no reference samples available for comparison to an unidentified individual or remains, then an identification may still be possible by searching any DNA profiles obtained against both national and international databases. In the United Kingdom, the UK National Criminal Intelligence DNA Database was established in 1995 and is used to store the profiles of men and women charged with crimes in England, Wales and Northern Ireland. A separate national DNA database is in operation in Scotland.

6.5.4 Incomplete and mixed profiles

6.5.4.1 *Incomplete profiles*

Due to sample degradation or the nature and size of an item itself, samples may yield insufficient DNA to produce a complete profile. In these instances an incomplete or partial profile may be obtained whereby components are not observed at all of the sites in a given test. In these instances, depending on the degree to which the profile is incomplete, it may still be possible to use such profiles to distinguish individuals or remains from each other and make meaningful comparisons to reference profiles. However, the statistical significance of these comparisons, and therefore the strength of the evidence derived from them, may be reduced to a greater or lesser extent dependent on the amount of information missing.

6.5.4.2   Mixed profiles

If remains have been commingled or best practice has not been followed in the collection, handling and processing of items, DNA from more than one source may be present in a sample. This can result in a mixed DNA profile whereby DNA from the two (or more) sources is visible in the result. Depending on the degree to which each individual has contributed to this mixture, it is sometimes possible to determine the DNA profiles of the individual contributors. However, in the case of both unidentified items and reference samples, this still causes difficulties in interpreting such results casting doubt as to which of the contributors an item genuinely relates to. In such instances, and where possible, it is therefore recommended that items are re-sampled or alternative items sought.

6.6   Conclusion

With regard to victim identification, DNA has been used since the 1990s and a number of methods exist and continue to be developed for victim identification and these have been stated above. Even when the deceased has not been identified by the different methods or by attempting to match his or her profile to DNA from missing persons, DNA may also provide some clues as to the biological profile of the individual including sex determination and ancestry.

Finally, the forensic scientist reporting the DNA results may be called to go to court as an expert witness.

References

Buckleton, J., Triggs, C. and Walsh, S. 2005. *Forensic DNA Interpretation*. CRC Press, Boca Raton, FL.

Butler, J.M. 2005. *Forensic DNA Typing*, 2nd edn. Elsevier/Academic Press, London.

Jeffreys, A., Wilson, V. and Thein, S. 1985. Individual-specific 'fingerprints' of human DNA. *Nature* **316**: 76–79.

7

Other scientific methods related to victim identification

7.1 Introduction

Nicholas Márquez-Grant[1] and Julie Roberts[2]
[1]Cellmark Forensic Services, Abingdon, UK; and Institute of Human Sciences, School of Anthropology and Museum Ethnography, University of Oxford, Oxford, UK
[2]Cellmark Forensic Services, Chorley, UK

On occasions the forensic anthropologist or other specialist may recommend further analysis to the Forensic Coordinator or SIO; for example if it has not been possible to establish whether remains are recent and of forensic interest, or whether they are archaeological. Dating of an isolated bone without much contextual information (e.g. a bone washed from the sea) may rely on techniques beyond that of an archaeological or anthropological assessment. This information is crucial in the investigation process and should contribute towards positive identification of the deceased. Likewise, it may not be possible to determine whether a bone fragment is human or non-human (animal) from macroscopic examination alone and microscopic, chemical or histological analysis may be required.

Since this volume is primarily concerned with the application of scientific techniques that can assist in death investigation and victim identification, a number of disciplines less commonly used and not strictly environmental in nature are described below. They are included as in our experience, when used alongside the disciplines and techniques described in other chapters, they have provided information which enabled a case to be resolved.

The first section, authored by Professor Gordon Cook, relates to dating techniques of bone that rely on chemical analysis of the bone itself. The second section, authored by Dr Sophie Beckett, relates to histological, isotope and other techniques which anthropologists and other scientists, as well as police officers, should be aware of.

Forensic Ecology Handbook: From Crime Scene to Court, First Edition.
Edited by Nicholas Márquez-Grant and Julie Roberts.
© 2012 John Wiley & Sons, Ltd. Published 2012 by John Wiley & Sons, Ltd.

7.2   Dating of human remains

Gordon Cook
Scottish Universities Environmental Research Group (SUERC), East Kilbride, Scotland, UK

Radiocarbon (^{14}C) dating is the most widely used technique for determining the age of human remains. Traditionally, the technique has been applied to the dating of bone and teeth samples of archaeological origin (between 300 and 50 000 years old approx.) but more recently it has been applied to equivalent samples from modern remains deriving from the latter half of the twentieth century to the present day.

7.2.1   How does radiocarbon dating work?

The archaeological application relies on the fact that ^{14}C is produced at a relatively constant rate in the upper atmosphere by the interaction of thermal neutrons with atmospheric nitrogen:

$$^{14}_{7}N + n \rightarrow {}^{14}_{6}C + p$$

The ^{14}C is rapidly oxidised to $^{14}CO_2$ which mixes quickly in the atmosphere with the stable forms of CO_2: $^{12}CO_2$ and $^{13}CO_2$. The CO_2 is taken up by plants during photosynthesis, thus labelling all plant life with ^{14}C as follows:

$$6CO_2 + 12H_2O \xrightarrow{\text{Light + chlorophyll}} C_6H_{12}O_6 + 6O_2 + 6H_2O$$

The plants are eaten by animals thus labelling all animal life with ^{14}C.

All of these processes are rapid with respect to the average lifetime of ^{14}C (8268 years). The average lifetime is distinct from the physical half-life of ^{14}C (5730 years). However, in radiocarbon dating the so-called Libby half-life of 5568 years is still used (this is explained later). As long as an organism is living, it retains what is termed an *equilibrium living value* of ^{14}C, for which the accepted value is 0.226 Bq g^{-1} of carbon. As soon as the organism dies, it ceases to exchange ^{14}C and so the level decreases in accordance with its half-life, decaying back to ^{14}N:

$$^{14}_{6}C \rightarrow {}^{14}_{7}N + \beta^-$$

The radiocarbon age (i.e. the time that has elapsed since the organism ceased to exchange carbon) is calculated according to the following equation:

$$t = \frac{1}{\lambda} \ln \left(\frac{A_o}{A_t} \right)$$

where t = time since carbon exchange ceased; λ = decay constant for ^{14}C = ln(2)/half-life = 0.693/5568 = 1.245×10^{-4} y^{-1}; A_0 = equilibrium living value of ^{14}C and A_t = activity t years after cessation of carbon exchange. The A_t value is measured in the laboratory. The A_0 value is the equilibrium living value and so cannot be measured directly. Its activity is estimated in the laboratory by measuring the activity of what is called the modern reference standard (SRM-4990C) whose activity is related to the theoretical A_0 value of 0.226 Bq g^{-1} C. This is based on the assumption that the equilibrium living value has been constant throughout the applied timescale of the ^{14}C dating method. In fact, this value has varied over the long term by a few percent but in radiocarbon dating, this is accounted for by what is called a calibration curve in which long sequences of known age samples (including annually formed tree rings, varved sediments and annually banded corals) are ^{14}C dated and their calendar ages plotted against their ^{14}C ages. This also corrects for the fact that in ^{14}C dating the so-called Libby half-life of 5568 years is still employed in age calculations rather than the true physical half-life of 5730 years.

With the onset of the Industrial Revolution there was massive burning of fossil fuels which resulted in the release of ^{12}CO$_2$ and ^{13}CO$_2$ into the atmosphere but because of their great age, all the ^{14}C had decayed and hence no ^{14}CO$_2$ was produced.

This resulted in dilution of ^{14}CO$_2$ in the atmosphere such that by 1890 AD, this effect was measurable in tree rings of that period. By the late 1940s, this had resulted in a 3 % reduction in the activity of ^{14}C in the atmosphere of the Northern Hemisphere (Suess, 1955). Then, in the 1950s and early 1960s, atmospheric nuclear weapons testing caused an almost doubling of the atmospheric ^{14}C activity of the Northern Hemisphere, while in the Southern Hemisphere the activity rose to around 1.67 times the natural level. In 1963 there was a partial test ban treaty and since then the ^{14}C activity in the atmosphere has declined as the excess enters the biota and the oceans. Figure 7.1 illustrates the atmospheric ^{14}C activity in the Northern Hemisphere between 1950 and 2010. These data are largely from measurements made on single tree rings whose ^{14}C activities are in equilibrium with the contemporaneous atmosphere (it is important to note that a tree ring only exchanges carbon during the year in which it is laid down). While these disturbances of the natural ^{14}C record have had an adverse influence on our ability to undertake radiocarbon dating of approximately post-1650 AD samples, the atmospheric nuclear weapons peak has provided us with a means of carrying out relatively precise age estimates on certain sample types that were formed post 1950 AD.

7.2.2 ^{14}C Dating of bone

For archaeological samples that have not been cremated it is the norm that the protein fraction (largely collagen) is dated. The hydroxyapatite (a form of calcium phosphate) component does contain a small carbonate component but this was deemed unsuitable for dating because of post-mortem exchange with inorganic carbon in the surrounding burial environment. In 1998, Lanting and Brindley

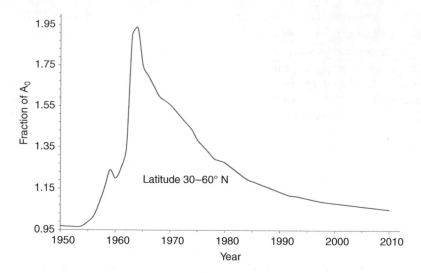

Figure 7.1 Variations in atmospheric ^{14}C as a consequence of atmospheric nuclear weapons testing. Courtesy of Gordon Cook/SUERC.

developed a technique for dating this carbonate fraction in cremated bones. The argument put forward for the success of this technique is that the cremation process locks in this carbonate component, preventing exchange (van Strydonck *et al.*, 2005).

Question: From a forensic perspective, what can we tell by dating collagen from recent bone samples where, in many instances, the extent of the human remains that are found may comprise only a single limb bone or a skull (quite often a cranium that is devoid of teeth)?

Answer: Basically, if the ^{14}C activity is above the natural level (0.226 Bq g^{-1} carbon) then the person definitely died during the nuclear era (last 50-odd years) and therefore there may be a requirement for further investigation. The reason that it is not possible (at least at present) to be more precise is because of the slow rate of collagen turnover in bones, particularly in adults. The turnover rate in an adult femoral mid-shaft has been estimated at <5 % yr^{-1}. It declines from approximately 4 % per annum to approximately 3 % per annum in females aged 20 to 80 years of age while male collagen turnover rates averaged 1.5–3 % per annum over the same period. During adolescent growth it is much higher (5–15 % yr^{-1} at age 10–15 years); however, the bone collagen ^{14}C activity is never in equilibrium with the atmosphere (Hedges *et al.*, 2007). The collagen activity at the time of death actually reflects some approximation to the average activity over the preceding 1–2 decades or even more. More research is undoubtedly required to gain a better understanding of the rate of collagen turnover in different bones and in people of different ages. Only when this is accomplished will there be the possibility of being able to apply ^{14}C measurements made on bone samples to make some sort of estimate of a person's year of birth.

7.2.3 ^{14}C Dating of teeth

When teeth are present, there is the potential to provide quite a precise estimate of the year of birth for people who were born during the nuclear era or directly prior to this time (up to approx. 55 years age). The reason lies in the fact that tooth enamel contains a small carbonate component (approx. 0.4 %) which does not exchange (Spalding *et al.*, 2005). The authors argue that the ^{14}C activity of the carbonate component is a reflection of the ^{14}C activity in the atmosphere during the time of enamel formation and of course, we know relatively precisely when the various teeth form in the body. Taking these points together with the fact that the activity in the atmosphere has been changing relatively rapidly over the past 50 years or so, this provides the ability to assign the measured ^{14}C activity to a specific year (or years) (Spalding *et al.*, 2005). This is contrary to earlier research showing that ^{14}C activities in human tissue (not teeth) were unlikely to mirror exactly the atmospheric trends (Harkness and Walton, 1969, 1972; Stenhouse and Baxter, 1977), although, a recent study by Hodgkins (2009) indicated that blood, hair and nail radiocarbon levels lagged atmospheric levels by only 0 to 3 years, consistent with a rapid replacement of these tissues.

The assumption of ^{14}C activities in tissues mirroring that of the contemporaneous atmosphere is quite valid for archaeological dating as the ^{14}C activity of the atmosphere is relatively constant. Also, typical errors on archaeological bone samples of Holocene age (approx. last 10 000 years) would be of the order of 25–50 years. However, the short timescales and high precision that Spalding *et al.* (2005) are dealing with, together with the fact that the ^{14}C activity in the atmosphere is changing relatively rapidly within the nuclear era, would seem to preclude the possibility of achieving equilibrium, particularly when diet (^{14}C turnover time in meat and the marine reservoir effect for marine resources) is taken into consideration. However, since tooth enamel is formed at a very young age, when children are actively growing and carbon turnover is rapid, the lag between tooth enamel and the contemporaneous atmosphere will be minimised and indeed the results of their study are quite convincing.

In cases where there is ambiguity (i.e. does the ^{14}C activity reflect a year when the activity was rising to the peak in 1963 or a year post-1963 when the activity was declining), this can be resolved by measuring the activity in teeth that form at different times after birth, for example by using a central incisor and a second molar. If the activity in the central incisor (for which crown formation is complete by 4–5 years after birth) is lower than that of the second molar (for which crown formation is complete by 7–8 years after birth), the year of birth is pre-1963, that is, on the upslope of the bomb ^{14}C peak. The opposite trend would apply for a post-1963 year of birth. A different approach that has been proposed is to measure the ^{14}C in crown enamel to establish the two age ranges, and ^{14}C in cortical and trabecular bone samples from the same skeleton to establish whether the age range was pre- or post-1963. This can be achieved because most trabecular bone undergoes faster collagen turnover than most cortical bone (Ubelaker, Buchholz and Stewart, 2006).

Work carried out in the SUERC ^{14}C laboratory has demonstrated that a single tooth can be used to unambiguously define the age (Cook *et al.*, 2006). This has been established by measuring the ^{14}C in the crown enamel, and the collagen-like component from the dentine and cementum from the root. Since the root forms after the crown, pre-1963 birth should be indicated by the root having the higher activity, and for a post-1963 birth the root activity should be lower than that of the crown. These techniques have been shown to be accurate to within 1–2 years (Cook *et al.*, 2006; Spalding *et al.*, 2005).

7.2.4   Other radionuclide techniques

Swift *et al.* (2001) carried out a range of analyses on both naturally occurring and man-made radionuclides in human skeletal material. For the man-made radionuclides, they observed that ^{239,240}Pu (Plutonium) was only detectable in those individuals who had died during the nuclear era and was below the limit of detection for those individuals who had died prior to the nuclear era. Similarly, ^{137}Cs was detectable in some individuals who had died during the nuclear era but was otherwise below detection limits.

In terms of the naturally occurring radionuclides: the uranium concentration decreased in an approximately linear fashion from around 700 μg kg^{-1} in bone samples that had short post-mortem intervals to approaching 0 μg kg^{-1} in individuals with post-mortem intervals of around 80 years. The authors (Swift *et al.*, 2001) observe that such a decrease is contrary to the observation of elevated uranium (U) concentrations in fossil bone and propose that the depletions in concentration may be related to hydrolysis during decay of soft tissue. An inverse relationship is also observed between the date of death and the ^{234}U/^{238}U ratio. Finally, they also demonstrated a correlation between ^{210}Po (Polonium) and time since death. These correlations are worthy of further study and in combination with the detail offered by ^{14}C could yield additional information.

7.2.5   Other ancillary techniques

In addition to the techniques described above, there are many other associated isotopic analyses that could be used to help in the identification of human remains (see also Section 7.3). These include analysis of the stable isotopes of carbon (^{13}C/^{12}C ratio i.e. δ^{13}C), nitrogen (^{15}N/^{14}N ratio, i.e. δ^{15}N) and sulphur (^{34}S/^{32}S ratio i.e. δ^{34}S) in bone collagen. High consumption of marine resources is usually accompanied by heavy δ^{13}C values although this can be misinterpreted if the person had a diet containing a C_4 plant component as C_4 plants have similar $\delta^{13}C$ values to marine resources (Pate, 1997). However, heavy values of both $\delta^{13}C$ and $\delta^{15}N$ are normally indicative of consumption of marine resources (Schoeninger and DeNiro, 1984; Müldner et al., 2009). Alkass et al. (2011) suggest that $\delta^{13}C$ measurements on tooth enamel can provide some information on the geographic origin of the person; however, this was based on a relatively small data set and while this might be generally true when comparing populations that are liable to have strikingly different diets, a $\delta^{13}C$ value for an individual will be difficult to interpret in terms of their geographic origin. The $\delta^{34}S$ value of bone collagen is a reflection of the isotopic composition of the diet which in turns reflects the geology of the food origin (Peterson, Howarth and Garritt, 1985).

Stable lead isotope ratios in tooth enamel have been used as historical biomarkers. For example, imported Australian ore, with a lower $^{206}Pb/^{207}Pb$ ratio (1.04) than native values from coal-burning and smelting activities (1.17–1.18), was used in the manufacture of alkyl lead additives for UK petrol from around 1930 until the end of the twentieth century (Farmer, MacKenzie and Moody, 2006). It may be possible to relate the decrease in the $^{206}Pb/^{207}Pb$ ratio, as the use of petrol lead increases, to a year or years when the tooth enamel was laid down.

Strontium ratios ($^{87}Sr/^{86}Sr$) in tooth enamel have been used to source a person's origin in archaeological populations (Budd et al., 2000; Müldner et al., 2009). Geographical variation in strontium isotopes is primarily controlled by the underlying geology but there are many other factors that need to be considered (Montgomery, 2010); although strontium analysis in bone from archaeological populations is considered unreliable because of post-mortem contamination or diagenesis of tissues in the burial environment (Budd et al., 2000). Harbeck et al. (2011) suggest that data from bones of modern individuals can provide hints to their geographic origin, even when the analyses are conducted on fully cremated bones. Finally, the stable isotope ratio of oxygen ($^{18}O/^{16}O$ ratios, i.e. $\delta^{18}O$) in tooth enamel phosphate or carbonate largely reflects the isotopic composition of drinking water, which in turn is usually equivalent to that of the local precipitation (Longinelli, 1984; Bryant and Froelich, 1995) and so it may provide some information on the geographic location of the person's origin.

All of the techniques described above have been applied quite widely to archaeological populations; however, in an era when we source our food and drink worldwide, significant research is undoubtedly required to establish whether those methods designed to establish geographic origin are suitable for forensic investigation of modern human remains.

References

Alkass, K., Buchholz, B.A., Druid, H. and Spalding, K.L. 2011. Analysis of ^{14}C and ^{13}C in teeth provides precise birth dating and clues to geographical origin. *Forensic Science International* **209**: 34–41.

Bryant, J.D. and Froelich, P.N. 1995. A model of oxygen isotope fractionation in body water of large mammals. *Geochimica et Cosmochimica Acta* **59**: 4523–4537.

Budd, P., Montgomery, J., Barriero, B. and Thomas, R.G. 2000. Differential diagenesis of strontium in archaeological human dental tissues. *Applied Geochemistry* **15**: 687–694.

Cook, G.T., Dunbar, E., Black, S.M. and Xu, S. 2006. A preliminary assessment of age at death determination using the nuclear weapons testing ^{14}C activity of dentine and enamel. *Radiocarbon* **48**: 305–313.

Farmer, J.G., MacKenzie, A.B. and Moody, G.H. 2006. Human teeth as historical biomonitors of environmental and dietary lead: some lessons from isotopic studies of 19th and 20th century archival material. *Environmental Geochemistry and Health* **28**: 421–430.

Harbeck, M., Schleuder, R., Schneider, J. *et al.* 2011. Research potential and limitations of trace analyses of cremated remains. *Forensic Science International* **204**: 191–200.

Harkness, D.D. and Walton, A. 1969. Carbon-14 in the biosphere and humans. *Nature* **223**: 1216–1218.

Harkness, D.D. and Walton, A. 1972. Further investigations of the transfer of bomb ^{14}C to man. *Nature* **240**: 302–303.

Hedges, R.E., Clement, J.G., Thomas, C.D. and O'Connell, T.C. 2007. Collagen turnover in the adult femoral mid-shaft: modeled from anthropogenic radiocarbon tracer measurements. *American Journal of Physical Anthropology* **133**: 808–816.

Hodgkins, G.W.L. 2009. *Measuring atomic bomb-derived ^{14}C levels in human remains to determine year of birth and/or year of death.* Report to the U.S. Department of Justice.

Lanting, J.N. and Brindley, A.L. 1998. Dating cremated bone: the dawn of a new era. *Journal of Irish Archaeology* **9**: 1–7.

Longinelli, A. 1984. Oxygen isotopes in mammal bone phosphate: a new tool for palaeohydrological and palaeoclimatological research. *Geochimica et Cosmochimica Acta* **48**: 385–390.

Montgomery, J. 2010. Passports from the past: Investigating human dispersals using strontium isotope analysis of tooth enamel. *Annals of Human Biology* **37**: 325–346.

Müldner, G., Montgomery, J., Cook, G. *et al.* 2009. The Bishops of Whithorn: Isotope evidence for status and mobility amongst medieval clerics in Scotland. *Antiquity* **83**: 1119–1133.

Pate, F.D. 1997. Bone chemistry and palaeodiet: Reconstructing prehistoric subsistence-settlement systems in Australia. *Journal of Anthropological Archaeology* **16**: 103–120.

Peterson, B.J., Howarth, R.W. and Garritt, R.H. 1985. Multiple stable isotopes used to trace the flow of organic matter in estuarine food webs. *Science* **227**: 1361–1363.

Schoeninger, M.J. and DeNiro, M.J. 1984. Nitrogen and carbon isotopic composition of bone collagen from marine and terrestrial mammals. *Geochimica et Cosmochimica Acta*, **48**: 625–639.

Spalding, K.L., Buchholz, B.A., Bergman, L.E. *et al.* 2005. Age written in teeth by nuclear tests. *Nature* **437**: 333–334.

Stenhouse, M.J. and Baxter, M.S. 1977. Bomb ^{14}C as a biological tracer. *Nature* **267**: 828–832.

Suess, H.E. 1955. Radiocarbon concentration in modern wood. *Science* **122**: 415–417.

Swift, B., Lauder, I., Black, S. and Norris, J. 2001. An estimation of the post-mortem interval in human skeletal remains: a radionuclide and trace element approach. *Forensic Science International* **117**: 73–87.

Ubelaker, D.H., Buchholz, B.A. and Stewart, J.E.B. 2006. Analysis of artificial radiocarbon in different skeletal and dental tissue types to evaluate date of death. *Journal of Forensic Science* **51**: 484–488.

van Strydonck, M., Boudin, M., Hoefens, M. and de Mulder, G. 2005. ^{14}C-dating of cremated bones – why does it work? *Lunula* **13**: 3–10.

7.3 Other analytical techniques

Sophie Beckett
Cranfield Forensic Institute, Cranfield University, Shrivenham, UK

A forensic anthropologist can confirm the presence of human skeletal remains at a crime scene and can provide a considerable amount of information from examination of the skeletal material in the mortuary, or laboratory (see Chapter 4). In some cases, it may be necessary to employ additional analytical techniques in order to answer key initial questions such as: 'Is it bone?', 'Is it human?' and 'Is it of forensic relevance?' Once positive answers have been established for these questions, the further application of analytical techniques can yield valuable intelligence for investigators.

The question of whether a piece of evidence is bone can often be readily determined by the use of radiography (see Chapter 5). This is a rapid and non-destructive tool that has the capability of answering several further questions. In addition, recent technological developments have enabled the exploration of the anthropological potentials of computed tomography (CT) and high resolution CT (micro-CT) as they become increasingly accessible laboratory techniques (Cooper, Thomas and Clement, 2011; O'Connell *et al.*, 2011). CT and micro-CT enable 3D reconstructions to be obtained from a series of 2D digital radiographs. They can be used to non-destructively examine the internal characteristics of a sample by digitally sectioning the reconstructed data. Regions of interest can also be highlighted by selective display based on material density. Micro-computed tomography is not yet able to offer the same level of structural resolution that can be obtained by use of histology but as this technique continues to be developed, it is hoped that this will be achieved in the near future. In the first instance, micro-CT can be applied to confirm the presence of material with internal structures consistent with bone (Reiche *et al.*, 2011) but has considerable capability beyond this. It is anticipated that CT scanning will become a routine approach to triaging and identification in disaster victim identification operations (O'Connell *et al.*, 2011) and both CT and micro-CT will make a significant contribution to many areas of forensic anthropology. Recent research has demonstrated the potential for the use of CT for age estimation (Bassed, Briggs and Drummer, 2010), sex estimation (Ramsthaler *et al.*, 2010) and micro-CT for trauma analysis (Robson Brown *et al.*, 2011; Sano *et al.*, 2011; see also Chapter 5).

In addition to the imaging techniques available, various applied chemistry techniques can be used to indicate the presence of bone material. X-ray diffraction (XRD) analysis, which provides information on the composition and (crystal) structure of crystalline materials, can confirm the presence of a form of calcium hydroxylapatite (bone mineral). X-ray fluorescence (XRF) analysis is used to determine elemental composition of a sample and can confirm the presence of elements consistent with bone mineral such as calcium and phosphorous. Each of these techniques can be of particular relevance when the microscopic architectural integrity of bone evidence has been compromised, for example in cases of burnt and/or powdered bone such as ashed remains.

When human or other animal origin of bone cannot be readily determined by the forensic anthropologist there are several analytical approaches that may be of assistance. DNA analysis can be used to confirm the presence of human bone. The use of this technique to determine human identity is discussed earlier in Chapter 6. However, DNA analysis is not always successful, especially in cases where DNA integrity of bone has been significantly affected by burning or diagenesis. Bone histology, which has been a valuable resource in forensic anthropology for many years, can be used to identify the microscopic internal structural features of bone (Stout and Crowder, 2011). It is a destructive 2D technique but one that can provide a wealth of information beyond simply identifying evidence as bone and it is therefore commonly employed for a range of purposes. It is often employed to assist in differentiating human from non-human bone but it is limited in its ability to determine species (Mulhern, 2009; Mulhern and Ubelaker, 2011).

Several biomolecular techniques have demonstrated, moreover, an ability to identify species from bone. One method uses matrix-assisted laser desorption/ionisation time-of-flight mass spectrometry (MALDI-TOF-MS) to analyse species-specific peptide markers extracted from bone collagen (Buckley *et al.*, 2009, 2010). Another method uses protein radio-immunoassay (pRIA) to test species-specific antibody responses to albumin within protein samples extracted from bone (Ubelaker, Lowenstein and Hood, 2004). Both techniques require only small (mg) samples but involve intricate chemistry protocols and may not be successful when the organic component of bone has been significantly degraded, for example through diagenesis or burning. An XRD approach that interrogates the inorganic component of bone has demonstrated its potential for species identification too (Beckett, Rogers and Clement, 2011). Although the application of XRD is destructive in this context, only small (mg) samples are needed and it is again of particular relevance in analysis of burnt bone fragments and ashes. The continued development of these techniques in the future may establish them as routine practical alternatives to DNA analysis.

Establishing whether human bone is of forensic relevance in terms of time-since-death can be achieved through the use of radiocarbon dating (see Section 7.2). Over many years, numerous other methods for estimating time-since-death have been investigated including histology, the analysis of nitrogen content in bone, XRD and Raman spectroscopy. However, none have been routinely adopted and there is still a need for current research to be carried out in this subject area (Forbes and Nugent, 2009; see Section 7.2). Once it has been established that a piece of evidence is human bone of forensic relevance, there are many subsequent lines of enquiry that can benefit from the use of analytical techniques, some of which are considered here. These include obtaining a biological profile of the deceased. Apart from the macroscopic or visual anthropological assessment of the human remains, age-at-death can be estimated through the application of bone histology but individual biological variation limits its accuracy and reliability (Crowder, 2009). Recent research has investigated the potential for radiocarbon dating (see Section 7.2) to also provide an estimation of age-at-death, with promising results (Lynnerup *et al.*, 2010; Ubelaker and Parra, 2011). Stable isotope analyses of bone have been used for many years in archaeological science and are now increasingly being applied to forensic cases to provide human geological provenancing and dietary intelligence. Stable isotopes of strontium, oxygen, carbon and nitrogen have each demonstrated their potential value to forensic investigation of bone and tooth evidence (Chenery *et al.*, 2010; Juarez, 2008; Meier-Augenstein, 2010).

In summary, a wide range of analytical techniques make a valuable contribution to the investigation of bone evidence in victim identification and forensic anthropology. Some are well established and are used routinely whilst others are rapidly demonstrating their potential and being increasingly employed in forensic cases. In most cases, a multi-technique approach can be advantageous and enable complementary information to be gained from the use of several different techniques. With each analytical approach adopted, it is important that: (a) it is question-led; (b) there is an understanding of the relevance of the techniques to the evidence under investigation and the limitations of each technique employed; and (c) that investigations are planned to ensure non-destructive methods are carried out prior to destructive analyses.

References

Bassed, R.B., Briggs, C. and Drummer, O.H. 2010. Analysis of time of closure of the spheno-occipital synchondrosis using computed tomography. *Forensic Science International* **200**: 161–164.

Beckett, S., Rogers, K.D. and Clement, J.G. 2011. Inter-species variation in bone mineral behavior upon heating. *Journal of Forensic Sciences* **56**: 571–579.

Buckley, M., Collins, M., Thomas-Oates, J. and Wilson, J.C. 2009. Species identification by analysis of bone collagen using matrix-assisted laser desorption/ionisation time-of-flight mass spectrometry. *Rapid Communications in Mass Spectrometry* **23**: 2843–3854.

Buckley, M., Collins, M., Thomas-Oates, J. and Wilson, J.C. 2010. Erratum: Species identification by analysis of bone collagen using matrix-assisted laser desorption/ionisation time-of-flight mass spectrometry. *Rapid Communications in Mass Spectrometry* **24**: 3372.

Chenery, C., Müldner, G., Evans, J. *et al.* 2010. Strontium and stable isotope evidence for diet and mobility in Roman Gloucester, UK. *Journal of Archaeological Science* **37**: 150–163.

Cooper, D.M.L., Thomas, C.D.L. and Clement, J.G. 2011. Technological developments in the analysis of cortical bone histology: the third dimension and its potential in anthropology. In C. Crowder and S. Stout (eds) *Bone Histology: An Anthropological Perspective*. CRC Press, Boca Raton, FL, pp. 361–375.

Crowder, C. 2009. Histological age estimation. In S. Blau and D.H. Ubelaker (eds) *Handbook of Forensic Anthropology and Archaeology*. Left Coast Press, Walnut Creek, CA, pp. 222–235.

Forbes, S. and Nugent, K. 2009. Dating of anthropological skeletal remains of forensic interest. In S. Blau and D.H. Ubelaker (eds) *Handbook of Forensic Anthropology and Archaeology*. Left Coast Press, Walnut Creek, CA, pp. 164–186.

Juarez, C.A. 2008. Strontium and geolocation, the pathway to identification for deceased undocumented Mexican border-crossers: A preliminary report. *Journal of Forensic Sciences* **53**: 46–49.

Lynnerup, N., Kjeldsen, H., Zweihoff, R. *et al.* 2010. Ascertaining year of birth/age at death in forensic cases: A review of conventional methods and methods allowing for absolute chronology. *Forensic Science International* **201**: 74–78.

Meier-Augenstein, W. 2010. *Stable Isotope Forensics: An Introduction to the Forensic Application of Stable Isotope Analysis*. John Wiley & Sons, Ltd, Chichester.

Mulhern, D.M. 2009. Differentiating human from non-human skeletal remains. In S. Blau and D.H. Ubelaker (eds) *Handbook of Forensic Anthropology and Archaeology*. Left Coast Press, Walnut Creek, CA, pp. 158–163.

Mulhern, D.M. and Ubelaker, D.H. 2011. Differentiating human from non-human bone microstructure. In C. Crowder and S. Stout (eds) *Bone Histology: An Anthropological Perspective*. CRC Press, Boca Raton, FL, pp. 109–134.

O'Connell, C., Lino, M., Mansharan, K. *et al.* 2011. Contribution of post-mortem multidetector CT scanning to identification of the deceased in a mass disaster: Experience gained from the 2009 Victorian bushfires. *Forensic Science International* **205**: 15–28.

Ramsthaler, R., Kettner, M., Gehl, A. and Verhoff, M.A. 2010. Digital forensic osteology: morphological sexing of skeletal remains using volume-rendered cranial CT scans. *Forensic Science International* **195**: 148–152.

Reiche, I., Muller, K., Staude, A. *et al.* 2011. Synchrotron radiation and laboratory micro X-ray computed tomography – useful tools for the material identification of prehistoric objects made of ivory, bone or antler. *Journal of Analytical Atomic Spectrometry* **26**: 1802–1812.

Robson Brown, K., Silver, I.A., Musgrave, J.H. and Roberts, A.M. 2011. The use of μCT technology to identify skull fracture in a case involving blunt force trauma. *Forensic Science International* **206**: e8–e11.

Sano, R., Hirawasa, S., Kobayashi, S. *et al.* 2011. Use of post-mortem computed tomography to reveal an intraoral gunshot injuries in a charred body. *Legal Medicine* **13**: 286–288.

Stout, S. and Crowder, C. 2011. Bone remodeling, histomorphology, and histomorphometry. In C. Crowder and S. Stout (eds) *Bone Histology: An Anthropological Perspective*. CRC Press, Boca Raton, FL, pp. 1–21.

Ubelaker, D.H. and Parra, R.C. 2011. Radiocarbon analysis of dental enamel and bone to evaluate date of birth and death: Perspective from the southern hemisphere. *Forensic Science International* **208**: 103–107.

Ubelaker, D.H., Lowenstein, J.M. and Hood, D.G. 2004. Use of solid-phase double-antibody radioimmunoassay to identify species from small skeletal fragments. *Journal of Forensic Sciences* **49**: 924–929.

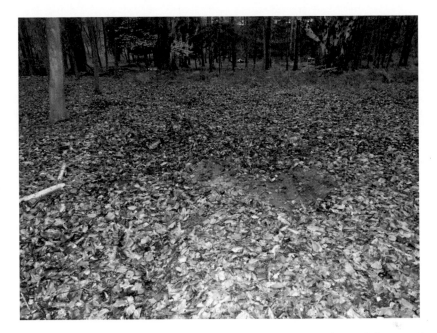

Plate 3.1 Potential target in the search of three clandestine graves in a training exercise. In this image, disturbed autumn surface vegetation layer and soil, and spoil is observed. Not clearly appreciated, but there is sinking of the ground and a number of tree stumps which potentially could serve as grave markers.

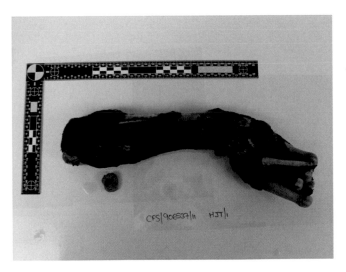

Plate 4.2 This 'body part' was submitted to the DNA laboratory as police thought it to be a human arm. On inspection by an anthropologist it was confirmed as non-human (it was in fact a seal limb). Courtesy of Cellmark Forensic Services.

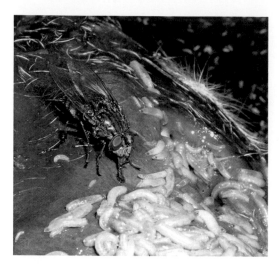

Plate 8.1   Bluebottle blowfly *Calliphora vicina,* surrounded by larvae of different sizes/ages.

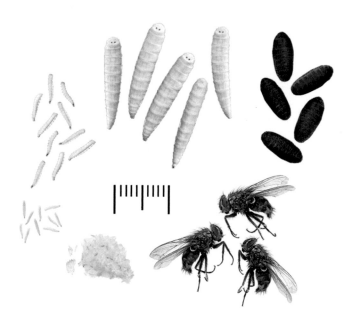

Plate 8.2   Life cycle of bluebottle blowfly *Calliphora vicina.* Clockwise from bottom left: eggs, 1st instar larvae, 2nd instar larvae, 3rd instar larvae, puparia (containing pupae), adult flies. Scale bar in millimetres.

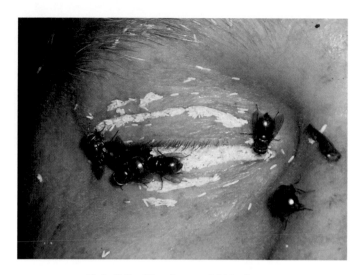

Plate 8.3 Blowfly eggs laid in the eye.

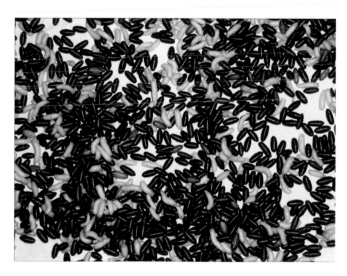

Plate 8.4 Post-feeding larvae (cream-coloured) and young (orange) and older (brown) puparia.

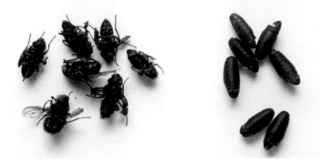

Plate 8.5 Adults with unextended wings (left), newly emerged from pupal cases (right).

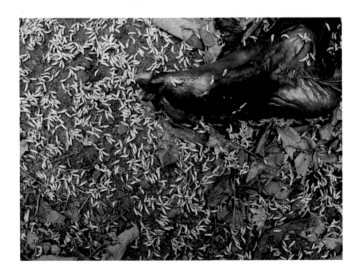

Plate 8.6 Post-feeding larvae dispersing from a body.

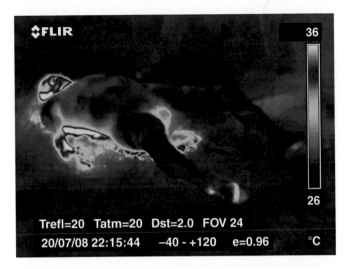

Plate 8.10 Infrared thermal image of human body showing increased temperatures at sites of larval masses, that is, on the head, the body–soil interface, and the anal-genital region.

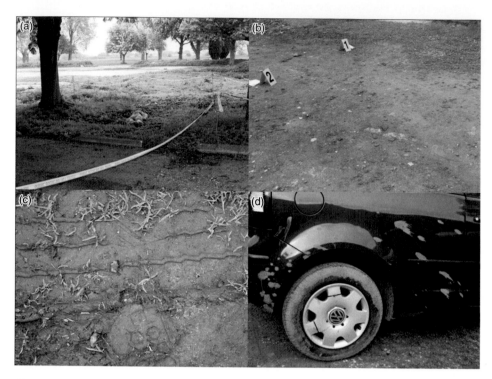

Plate 12.1 Soil sampling in forensic geology investigations. (a) With a surface body deposition, soil samples should be collected around the victim, taking into account the likely way in which the body was moved by the offender(s). In this case samples would also be taken from the adjacent road. Image courtesy of Manlove Forensics training course. (b) Areas such as this loosely surfaced car park can be very distinctive geologically because of the mix of both naturally occurring soils and introduced materials such as aggregates. (c) Where there are distinct vehicle tracks or footwear impressions, soil samples can either be taken from the impression itself or from a cast of the impression. (d) When sampling vehicles and other exhibits, the primary aim is to identify discrete depositional events; in this case the obvious mud splashes on the bodywork of a vehicle.

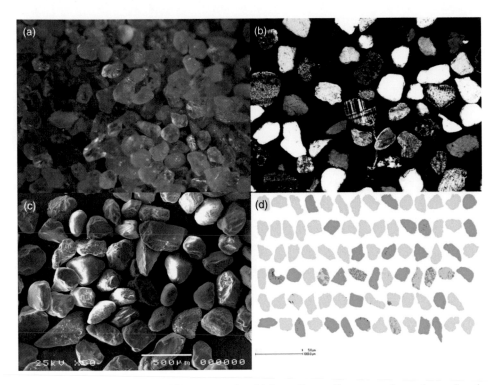

Plate 12.2 There are many different ways in which a soil or sediment sample can be analysed. In this case a sand sample collected from the Omaha D-Day landing beach is imaged: (a) using a binocular microscope, (b) under transmitted light microscopy following the preparation of a sand sample as a thin slice, (c) under manual scanning electron microscopy, and (d) as false colour images of mineral grains identified using automated scanning electron microscopy (QEMSCAN®) analysis; each colour represents a different mineral type.

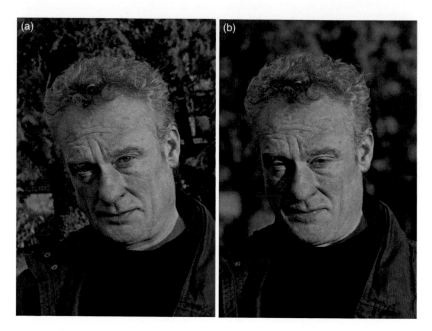

Plate 14.2 When taking a portrait image of a person, selecting a larger aperture will draw the viewer's attention to the subject and cause a blurring effect to the background behind. In image (a) the aperture is set at $f22$ and in (b) at $f5.6$.

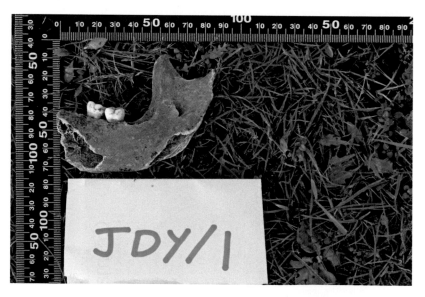

Plate 14.6 Digital images of crime scene items are disclosable to the court and should be recorded as they were on arrival and before they are moved in any way.

8

Forensic entomology

Martin Hall, Amoret Whitaker and Cameron Richards
Department of Life Sciences, Natural History Museum, London, UK

8.1 Introduction and current state of the discipline

Forensic entomology is the study of insects and other arthropods in a legal context (Hall, 2001), which can be broadly divided into three main areas of application (Lord and Stevenson, 1986): urban entomology (e.g. civil actions relating to insects and human environments), stored products entomology (e.g. civil actions relating to insects found in food products), and medico-legal entomology (e.g. criminal proceedings in cases of violent crime or unexpected death). The latter, sometimes also referred to as medico-criminal entomology (Hall, 1990), is the most high profile area of forensic entomology and the subject of this chapter. It can be utilised in many situations, from isolated domestic incidents to large-scale atrocity crimes, and for many different types of investigation: neglect of people in care, such as the elderly (Benecke, 2004); child abuse (Benecke and Lessig, 2001); wildlife poaching (Anderson, 1999; Samuel, 1988); detection of gunshot residue (Roeterdink, Dadour and Watling, 2004); detection of drugs, also called entomotoxicology (de Carvalho, 2010); movement of vehicles through identification of insects impacted on windscreens; transport and relocation of human remains (Smith, 1986); and estimation of minimum time-since-death (Hart, Whitaker and Hall, 2008).

Insects are ubiquitous in nature and it is almost inevitable that they will be associated with a crime scene, either because it is a part of their natural habitat or because they have been introduced or attracted to it. Since publication of the first manual of forensic entomology (Smith, 1986) there has been a surge of interest in the subject and major efforts have been made to increase the robustness of the interpretation of insect evidence. These activities have been reviewed extensively (Amendt *et al.*, 2010; Byrd and Castner, 2009; Haskell and Williams, 2008; Erzinçlioğlu, 2000; Gennard, 2007; Goff, 2000; Greenberg and Kunich, 2002).

The insects associated with human cadavers belong to one of four ecological groups: necrophagous species (feeding on the body); predators and parasites (of the necrophagous species); omnivorous species (feeding on the body and its

Forensic Ecology Handbook: From Crime Scene to Court, First Edition.
Edited by Nicholas Márquez-Grant and Julie Roberts.
© 2012 John Wiley & Sons, Ltd. Published 2012 by John Wiley & Sons, Ltd.

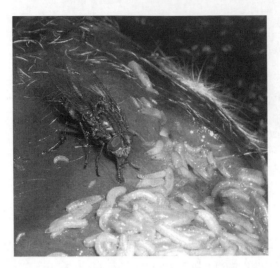

Figure 8.1   Bluebottle blowfly *Calliphora vicina,* surrounded by larvae of different sizes/ages. (To see a colour version of this figure, please see Plate 8.1.)

inhabitants); and adventive species (using the body as an extension of their environment) (Smith, 1986). The necrophagous species provide the information of greatest evidential value because of their direct and obligatory association with the body. Of greatest forensic importance in this group are the blowflies (Diptera: Calliphoridae) (Figure 8.1) because they are usually the first group to colonise a body and are found in greatest numbers, consequently they can provide the most accurate information regarding the minimum time-since-death (Greenberg, 1991). Blowflies have four developmental stages: egg, larva (maggot), pupa and adult (Figure 8.2). The larva is the main feeding stage and it passes through three instars (1st, 2nd and 3rd) which are separated by a moult (shedding) of the cuticle (skin) allowing for growth. Once larvae have finished feeding they move off the body and burrow into the soil, if outdoors, or under furniture and carpets, if indoors. Metamorphosis from larva to adult fly occurs during the pupal stage which takes place within the puparium, the hardened and darkened cuticle of the 3rd instar larva. In addition to blowflies, other insects collected from a body can have value in estimating a minimum time-since-death if their development rates are known, for example species of hide beetle (*Dermestes*) which are common on dried bodies (Kumara *et al.*, 2009; Midgley, Richards and Villet, 2010).

'When did the victim die?' can be a crucial question in cases of untimely death (Wells and Lamotte, 2001) and the estimation of time-since-death, also referred to as post-mortem interval (PMI), is the most frequent task required of a forensic entomologist. Of course what an entomologist actually establishes is the time of colonisation of a body by the insects that arrived first. This is, therefore, termed the minimum PMI (PMI$_{min}$) because there could be many reasons for a delay in colonisation (see Section 8.6.5). Many other methods have been applied to establish

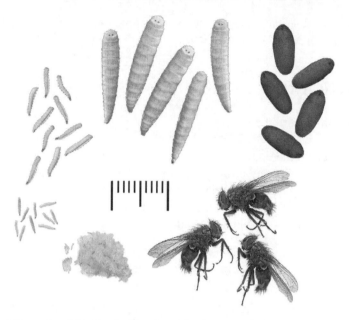

Figure 8.2   Life cycle of bluebottle blowfly *Calliphora vicina*. Clockwise from bottom left: eggs, 1st instar larvae, 2nd instar larvae, 3rd instar larvae, puparia (containing pupae), adult flies. Scale bar in millimetres. (To see a colour version of this figure, please see Plate 8.2.)

time-since-death, such as chemical, histological and bacteriological (Easton and Smith, 1970). However, most post-mortem changes in a cadaver measured by pathologists to estimate PMI (e.g. rigor mortis, algor mortis, livor mortis) are not reliable because of the inability to accurately account for the variability in these processes, and the reliance upon subjective evaluation rather than objective measurement (Henssge, Madea and Gallenkemper, 1988). In addition, most post-mortem changes used to estimate PMI occur within the first 72 hours of death, so the medical examiner's estimate is limited to these first three days. Swift (2010) concluded that, 'It remains debateable whether there is any single, reliable and accurate means of estimating the time since death during the early post-mortem interval' (p. 107).

Nevertheless, the first blowflies to lay eggs on a body start a biological clock ticking so that, using objective methods to study the colonisation and development of these insects, the time of death can be estimated over periods of a few weeks in summer and a few months in cooler seasons. If the discovery of a body is delayed beyond this period then the succeeding colonisers (mainly flies and beetles) will still provide a useful but less accurate time of death (Greenberg and Kunich, 2002). This is done by interpreting the changes in insect fauna composition that accompany decompositional changes. Insect succession was first observed by Mégnin (1894) and is now the subject of much research (e.g. Matuszewski *et al.*, 2011). However, it can be difficult to interpret and is subject to considerable local and seasonal variation, therefore it will not be considered in detail here. Measurement of changes in the chemical composition of empty puparia over time might become another tool in estimating longer PMIs (Drijfhout, 2010).

8.2 Applications

8.2.1 Introduction

As indicated above, there are many diverse applications for forensic entomology. Even the absence of insects on a body can be of value, for example confirming that a concealed body had not been exposed to fly activity before concealment (Erzinçlioğlu, 1996). However, the main applications relate to insect infestation or colonisation of living or dead humans and animals.

8.2.2 Live bodies

When fly larvae develop on living humans or other vertebrates they cause a disease condition known as myiasis (Hall and Smith, 1993; Hall and Wall, 1995). Although some species of myiasis-causing flies are obligatory parasites and cannot develop on dead animals, the majority of fly species associated with myiasis in a forensic context are the same species as are found on dead bodies. On live hosts they feed mainly on dead tissues within sites of trauma that have been neglected. Usually that neglect occurs in a domestic situation with either young children (e.g. as a result of soiled nappies) or the elderly (e.g. in infested bed sores). Occasionally neglect can occur even in a hospital or other medical environment leading to a hospital acquired (nosocomial) infestation. One example is that of a young boy who was admitted to hospital in a coma following a traffic accident. The emergence of two- to three-day-old larvae of the greenbottle blowfly *Lucilia sericata* from his nostrils four and five days after admission was consistent with infestation within the hospital (Hira *et al.*, 2004). In addition to being evidence of neglect in live humans and animals, myiasis infestations can cause problems in estimating PMI_{min} if overlooked. For example, if a victim of myiasis dies but it is assumed that the larval infestation began only after death, then the PMI_{min} estimate will be greater than it actually is. This can be shown by reference to a case in the United Kingdom, when the body of a woman was found indoors infested by large numbers of blowfly larvae, mostly dispersing from pressure sores in the anal region and thighs. The pathologist estimated that death had occurred about one day before collection of the larvae, but these were estimated by the entomologist to be two to three days old. The conclusion of an ante-mortem infestation was supported by the observation of a complete absence of any eggs or larvae in the exposed head orifices, where blowfly eggs are normally first laid. This ante-mortem myiasis infestation was, therefore, evidence of neglect by the carers of the deceased. Similar infestations of animals can be used as evidence of cruelty or neglect (Anderson and Huitson, 2004). For example, a case of infestation of the wound created by a wire snare around the neck of a trapped but still living badger in Scotland, with larvae estimated to be two to three days old, showed that the person who had set the snare had neglected to check it at least every day as was required by law.

8.2.3 Dead bodies

The major objective of a forensic entomology investigation is to determine the PMI_{min}. However, insect evidence can also help to indicate the manner of death (e.g. by directing a pathologist to knife wounds on bones below larval infested tissues in which any knife marks had been obliterated by larval feeding activity), the place of death and post-mortem movements of the body (e.g. through a knowledge of insect distribution and finding larvae on a body that were of a species not found in the locality of recovery), and can assist in toxicology studies when the body tissues are too degraded for analysis, that is, the larvae act as a reservoir for drugs in tissues they ingest (de Carvalho, 2010).

The value of insects in providing a PMI_{min} is exemplified by a case presented by Hart *et al.* (2008) in which the body of a young man was found behind a building in northern England in mid February. He had last been seen alive the previous November but pathology tests suggested he had been dead for just two weeks. However, aware of the potential for forensic entomology the pathologist asked for the insect evidence to be analysed. This gave a PMI_{min} consistent with death having occurred soon after the last sighting of the deceased. The body had lain in a shaded trench behind the building since death and the low winter temperatures had markedly slowed the rate of decomposition leading to the pathologist's underestimate of PMI. The low temperatures had also slowed the rate of insect development, but this was accounted for in estimating the PMI_{min} using forensic entomology techniques.

8.3 Pre-scene attendance

8.3.1 Information required pre-scene attendance

The forensic entomologist is generally notified by telephone that a body has been found and that their involvement is required. On some occasions, the Senior Investigating Officer (SIO) or Crime Scene Investigator (CSI) simply wants advice as to whether or not a forensic entomologist is actually required at the scene and, if not, how to collect the samples. In these situations, it is important to glean as much information about the scene and situation of the body as possible, and to provide instructions in a clear and concise manner. If it is possible for photographs of the body and scene, preferably prior to recovery, to be e-mailed to the forensic entomologist, this can help to give a clearer picture of the case.

However, attendance of a forensic entomologist at the scene or mortuary is often required to ensure an accurate evaluation and collection of the entomological evidence, in particular to ensure that the most relevant insect evidence is collected in an appropriate manner. If the body is discovered late in the day, attendance may be requested for the following day, but often the request is urgent and the entomologist is asked to attend as soon as possible, so that the body can be examined *in situ* prior to its removal from the scene. It is therefore advisable to have the entomological sampling equipment ready prepared and able to be accessed at short notice.

The first question to be asked of the SIO, CSI or Crime Scene Manager (CSM), is whether the body is indoors or outdoors, as additional equipment and clothing will be needed if the body is in an outdoor environment. An indication of the state of decomposition of the body and what insect activity is visible provides information on what might need to be collected so that preparations can be made before arrival at the scene. Ideally, early attendance at the scene of recovery of the body is preferable, to ensure that the insect evidence has not been disturbed so, if possible, a request should be made to the CSM not to move the body until the entomologist is in attendance.

8.3.2 Preparation pre-attendance

A clean, solid toolbox should be prepared and stored ready for use with the following recommended equipment:

- Forceps of varying sizes, both pliable and firm.
- Teaspoon (for collecting larvae when abundant).
- Sealable and aerated storage tubes of varying sizes (e.g. 10 ml, 30 ml, 50 ml, 150 ml).
- Specimen labels.
- 80 % ethanol (ethyl alcohol).
- Small sieve.
- Hand-held insect capture net.
- Protective clothing: disposable suits, gloves, shoe covers, facemasks.
- Disinfectant wipes and gel.
- Tape measure.
- Notebook, pens and pencils.
- Tin/pouch of moist dog food.
- Digital camera.

- Measuring scale for inclusion in photographic images.

- Hand-held infra-red and/or probe digital thermometer (calibrated and certified).

- Two electronic temperature dataloggers (calibrated and certified).

- Cooler bag and ice packs for live specimen transport.

Ethanol ($\geq 80\%$) is recommended as a preservative because, compared to most other preservatives such as formalin, it has relatively few health and safety concerns, it does not degrade DNA (analysis of which might be required) and it has less impact on the physical appearance of the samples (Adams and Hall, 2003). Additional equipment needed for outdoor scenes includes:

- Trowel.

- Plastic basin.

- Large soil sieve.

- Plastic sheet, e.g. 2 m $\times$ 2 m (to search soil samples on).

- Strong resealable bags, e.g. 25 cm $\times$ 35 cm (for holding soil samples).

- Stevenson screen (to protect datalogger from direct sunlight).

- Crime scene indicator flags.

- Compass or hand-held GPS.

Prior to attendance at the scene, two electronic dataloggers should be pre-set to record temperatures to match local weather station recording intervals (usually at hourly intervals, on the hour). More information regarding temperature recording is given in Section 8.6.4.

8.4 Scene attendance

8.4.1 Sampling protocols

Before proceeding with the collection of insect evidence, clear agreement for a sampling strategy should be reached with the CSM, pathologist and other forensic experts present at the scene to minimise the risk of inadvertently disturbing or destroying other evidence. Detailed and widely accepted protocols for sampling insect evidence have been published (Amendt *et al.*, 2007; Catts and Haskell, 1990) and are summarised here, with emphasis given to potential problems that can arise from common sampling errors made by untrained investigators, especially due to the lack of recognition of insect evidence, suboptimal sample size and incorrect labelling, handling and preservation. It is imperative that entomological evidence is collected

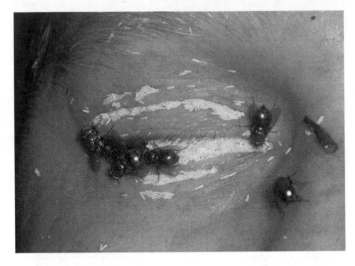

Figure 8.3   Blowfly eggs laid in the eye. (To see a colour version of this figure, please see Plate 8.3.)

in the correct manner, otherwise its value will be compromised and an accurate analysis will not be possible.

8.4.1.1   Sampling from the body

Insect eggs are at risk of predation and desiccation and are therefore usually laid at sites which minimise this, and where hatched larvae can gain ready access to soft tissues. In the majority of cases, blowfly eggs are first laid in and around the body orifices, usually beginning around the head, particularly in the mouth, nose, eyes and ears (Figure 8.3) and then the genital and rectal area if accessible. The body-soil interface and the scalp are also common sites for egg-laying. Eggs may also be concentrated at sites of trauma, for example where there are knife or gunshot wounds, and their location in such circumstances might provide information on the manner of death. Eggs can also be laid on clothing, especially in folds away from direct sunlight and if contaminated with blood or other body fluids. Eggs are fragile but can be collected without damage by using a fine paint brush or fine forceps, especially when they occur in large masses.

Larvae can be readily collected using pliable forceps or a small spoon, taking care not to inflict post-mortem wounds on the body of the deceased. It is important to record the sites from where larvae were collected. Specimens from different sites should not be combined but should be stored separately with detailed labelling. Records can be enhanced by photography of the sites of collection, ideally including a measurement scale, calibrated in mm.

It is essential to collect a sample of larvae for analysis that accurately reflects their abundance and diversity on the body (Hall *et al.*, 2008), that is, 50–100 larvae from each sample site. Although the entomologist is generally most concerned with the oldest insects, which are often the largest visible larvae, it is important to collect an accurate subset of all larvae. On occasion there may be a small number of larvae that appear to be significantly bigger than others – this could be due to their being precocious larvae, that is, having been laid as a 1st instar larva instead of as an egg (Wells and King, 2001), or their development may have been accelerated significantly, for example by feeding on tissues that were contaminated with drugs (Lord, 1990). Also, different species of fly may be present in the same larval mass, for instance many Sarcophagid (fleshfly) larvae are generally larger than blowfly larvae of the same age; conversely, the small larvae of some muscid species (e.g. the housefly, *Musca domestica*) could be older than the larger blowfly larvae. Therefore a sample should be collected that is representative of the complete range of larval sizes – a sample of six larvae from a mass of thousands will not provide confidence in PMI estimations.

Most people will easily recognise a writhing mass of larvae, but some life-stages of blowfly are more difficult to see, or if not moving, they may not be recognised as being of insect origin. Blowfly eggs are very small, about 1.5–3 mm long, immobile and are generally laid in dark and hidden areas such as the nose, mouth, ears, eyes, scalp and folds of the clothes as discussed above, and therefore may easily be overlooked (Figure 8.3). Likewise, as larvae enter the pupal stage they contract, harden and become dark brown and immobile (Figure 8.4), so they may also be overlooked, especially as they are often found some distance from the body. Therefore the possibility that the oldest specimens might have dispersed from the body should be considered (see Section 8.4.1.2). If adult flies have emerged, the empty pupal cases will remain in the environment as evidence of completed immature development (Figure 8.5) and these can also be easily overlooked resulting in an underestimate of PMI_{min} if only the younger larvae or unemerged puparia are collected.

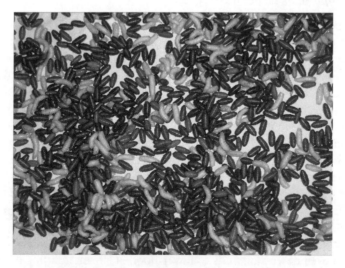

Figure 8.4 Post-feeding larvae (white) and young (pale) and older (dark) puparia. (To see a colour version of this figure, please see Plate 8.4.)

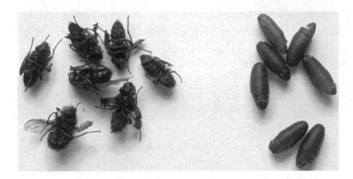

Figure 8.5   Adults with unextended wings (left), newly emerged from pupal cases (right). (To see a colour version of this figure, please see Plate 8.5.)

The insect fauna on a buried body may differ from that found on an exposed body (Payne, King and Beinhart, 1968), but collection of specimens from a buried body should proceed in a similar way to those described above, with a careful assessment of the layers of soil above, around and below the body to identify any evidence of insects moving towards or away from the body. While even a shallow burial (10–20 cm depth depending on soil texture) will deter most blowfly species, other groups of fly are more adept at colonising buried bodies. Species of *Muscina* (Diptera: Muscidae) (Gunn and Bird, 2011) and *Eumacronychia persolla* (Diptera: Sarcophagidae) (Szpila, Voss and Pape, 2010) will colonise bodies in shallow graves and species of scuttle flies (Phoridae) will colonise bodies buried under 1–2 m of soil (Disney, 1994; Gaudry, 2010).

8.4.1.2   Sampling of dispersed stages

During the post-feeding stage the larvae of most blowfly species leave the body (Figure 8.6) and search for a suitable pupariation site (Greenberg, 1991). If outdoors, larvae may disperse some distance from the body and then burrow down into the soil or under logs, stones and other ground cover. Therefore a search for dispersed insects should be conducted at several compass positions up to 5 m from the body, using a trowel to sample soil to a depth of about 15 cm. Care should be taken to exclude potential competing sources of larvae (e.g. dead wildlife) and control samples should be taken 10–20 m from the body to determine the background level of insect activity in the soil. Soil can be sieved and searched on a plastic sheet at the scene or can be bagged for inspection later in the laboratory.

At indoor scenes, dispersing larvae may be found under furniture and rugs, especially around the edge of the room, and even in rooms adjacent to that in which the body was found. On hard floors they can disperse much further than on soils and in blocks of flats larvae have been recorded to disperse under doors, into communal corridors and even down stairwells to lower floors. Care should therefore be taken to search some distance from the body.

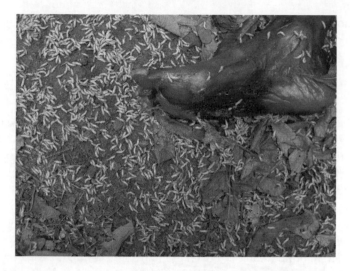

Figure 8.6   Post-feeding larvae dispersing from a body. (To see a colour version of this figure, please see Plate 8.6.)

8.4.1.3   *Handling of samples after collection*

Samples should be collected in two main batches:

- those to be killed and preserved at the time of collection to provide a record of the age of the insects at the time of collection (see Section 8.4.1.4);

- those to be kept alive for transport to the laboratory where they can be sub-sampled, some to be reared to the adult stage (see Section 8.6.1) and, where needed, some to be frozen for toxicological analysis and others to be frozen or preserved in ethanol for molecular studies, of both insect and human DNA (Wells *et al.*, 2001).

Eggs, larvae and pupae are living organisms and therefore they need to respire, so they should be placed in aerated sample tubes. These can be purchased or made simply by punching holes in lids, or by putting gauze or thick tissue held in place by elastic bands over standard specimen tubes, ensuring that the insects inside (such as small larvae) cannot escape through any openings. Also, if the larvae have been collected directly off the body it is likely that they are still feeding and therefore need a food source in the transport container in order to continue to develop. It is best to use the same food as that used in experiments that generated the development data being used for analysis. This is often liver, but if that is not available then alternatives such as minced meat or canned moist dog food should be used. In addition, live insects will die if they become either too cold or too hot, so they should not be placed in a freezer or left in a hot environment such as the boot of a car.

Ideally the samples should be placed in a cool bag for transport to the laboratory. If they need to be stored for a short period (ideally no more than 24 hours) then they should be kept in a fridge or left at room temperature with a temperature datalogger or some other record of their temperature (e.g. a simple thermometer will suffice).

8.4.1.4 Correct preservation

If fly larvae are not killed and preserved in the correct manner, their physical shape (length, curvature) will be changed which will make diagnostic characters difficult to see and affect the analysis to be carried out (Tantawi and Greenberg, 1993; Adams and Hall, 2003). Larvae placed directly into a tube without preservative will die and rapidly start to decompose or dehydrate making them difficult to analyse even soon afterwards, whereas samples properly preserved will retain their evidential value for many years (Figure 8.7). Eggs can be placed directly into 80 % ethanol. However, larvae will shrink in size if placed live into ethanol, so they need to be first killed in boiled water ($\geq 80°$C) by immersion for up to 30 seconds, before being sieved out and placed into ethanol. This will produce good-quality specimens, but if the immersion period is too short or the water not sufficiently hot, then preservation will be poor, resulting in deformed and discoloured larvae. The time and date of killing and preservation should be recorded. It is sometimes difficult to obtain boiled water at a crime scene, but this can usually be taken in a thermos flask or fetched from a catering van, a local cafe/restaurant, or from a nearby house. If ethanol is not available, a spirit such as vodka (*c.* 40–50 % alcohol) can be used instead, as long as this is noted and the samples are transferred into 80 % ethanol at the first opportunity.

Ideally, puparia should be killed in hot water prior to immersion in ethanol, but if hot water is not available, the cuticle of live puparia should be pricked to enable preservatives to penetrate readily. There is evidence that if not killed first, development of puparia can continue for some hours in ethanol (Richards, unpublished) – they can also survive for up to four days in water (Singh and Greenberg, 1994) – resulting in an incorrect estimate of PMI_{min}.

Any adult insects collected at the scene can be killed in the laboratory by placing into a deep freezer for one or more hours. After thawing they can be pinned for taxonomic study or stored in 80 % ethanol. Dried insects are very fragile and, if not pinned, are easily damaged when stored in bulk, losing hairs, wings and legs. Dead adults stored in humid conditions that prevent them drying will quickly decompose. For long-term storage dried insects should be stored in insect proof containers to prevent destruction by small beetles that feed on dead insects (e.g. museum or carpet beetles, *Anthrenus* species).

8.4.1.5 Correct labelling

It is important that samples are correctly labelled so that their provenance is known. Ideally, a label should be placed inside the tube with the preserved samples, written in pencil or archival quality micro-pigment inks, because most pen inks will

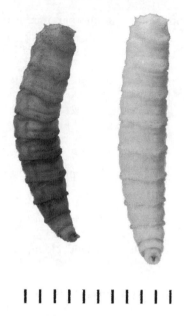

Figure 8.7 Blowfly larvae in 80 % ethanol, preserved badly (left – by immersion while still alive) and correctly (right – by first killing in hot water).

dissolve in ethanol. A label should also be attached to the outside of the container in both preserved and live samples. Information contained on the label should include: case name/location, police force or other client identifier, date, time of collection, where on the body or environment the insects were collected from, who collected the sample, and a unique sample number (the latter two are often combined). Examples are given below:

High St, Brentford 12th July 10 13:15 Inside shoe under bed APW/03	Operation Maggot July 12 2010 13:15 Scene/left nostril APW/05	Met Police/Brentford 12/07/10 at 1:15 pm Mortuary/right sock APW/10

8.4.2 Recording at the scene

Comprehensive notes should be taken during scene attendance to aid in preparing the final report. Details should be taken of date and time of attendance, location and a list of names and roles of all other people at the scene, including the pathologist, CSM, SIO, police photographer and any other forensic experts. It is also useful to exchange contact details with all these people in case you wish to communicate at a later date regarding the case.

Comprehensive notes and supporting photographs, if possible, should be taken regarding the scene:

- Indoor/outdoor.

- Rural/residential.

If indoor:

- Flat/house/shed or other description of the property.

- Curtains/windows/doors – open/closed/ajar.

- Number of rooms/floors.

- What room the body is in; its state (furnished, clean, littered); is the body exposed to direct sunlight or not?

- What other potential larval food sources are available, e.g. meat pies, dog food?

If outdoor:

- Environment, e.g. woodland/field/road/water.

- Local flora, e.g. trees, shrubs, grassy with identifications if possible.

- Soil type, e.g. clay, chalky.

- Aspect, e.g. shaded, exposed to sun.

Comprehensive notes should be taken regarding the body:

- Male/female.
- State of decomposition, e.g. fresh, bloat, active decay, advanced decay, dry/skeletal (Anderson and VanLaerhoven, 1996).
- Clothed/semi-clothed/naked.
- Wounds and their locations, e.g. knife, gunshot.
- Position, e.g. lying/sitting/hunched, face up/down.
- Direction of body, e.g. head facing north/south/east/west.
- Substrate, i.e. what is the body lying on?
- Contaminants/toxins – are any present on or in the body that could affect insect development?

An example of a scene/mortuary attendance form is provided in the Appendix to this chapter (based on Amendt *et al.*, 2007) and has a useful body outline diagram on which the location of insect evidence can be recorded.

In addition to collecting insect evidence, temperatures should be recorded at the scene and mortuary (if attended – see Section 8.5) of air, ground, body (on, in and under the corpse) and larval masses. A temperature probe may be used, but as this may cause the mass to disperse, the use of a non-invasive infra-red thermometer is recommended.

8.5 Mortuary attendance

Often a request is made to visit the mortuary and/or attend the post-mortem examination or autopsy. This may occur if the body was removed from the scene prior to the entomologist being called, or even after scene attendance, for instance if the body was removed before all sampling was completed. Movement of the body during its recovery can provoke larvae to disperse from their feeding sites and so present a distorted picture of the larval infestation when viewed at post-mortem. Therefore, although it is usually easier to collect insect samples directly from the body in the mortuary, scene attendance is still recommended so that insects can be collected from the body prior to disturbance, and also from the surrounding environment.

In the mortuary, it is important to follow instructions from the forensic pathologist and the mortuary technicians. If the body is clothed or wrapped, insect samples should be taken as it is being undressed or unwrapped to ensure that any important evidence is not lost. A record should be kept of where the samples are collected from.

It is important to record details of the mortuary temperature and, if used, that of its cold storage facility so that a record of temperatures to which the insect evidence was exposed is kept. This is because development of blowflies can be effectively suspended at the low temperatures (3–4°C) commonly found in mortuary cold stores (Johl and Anderson, 1996), although this effect will be less pronounced in a large larval mass. The mortuary technician will usually have details of mortuary temperatures together with the dates and times when the body was taken from one environment into another. In short, it is important to obtain the full 'thermal history' of the body including periods of transport and storage.

8.6 Laboratory analysis

8.6.1 Rearing of insect evidence

Live insect evidence is collected for rearing in a laboratory incubator for two principle reasons. Firstly, adult insects are easier to identify than larvae, so it is a useful way of confirming the identifications of the preserved immature stages. Secondly, if the insects are reared through at a known temperature, this thermal input can be subtracted from their known total developmental needs in order to ascertain how long they had been developing prior to collection, hence when they were deposited as eggs on the cadaver. This estimate of PMI_{min} can provide support to that calculated from larvae killed at the time of collection.

Insects should be reared through to adults in an incubator, set to a known constant temperature. If the temperature is too cool, the insects will take a long time to develop which might be critical if there are deadlines in the investigation to meet. On the other hand, if the temperature is too warm, the larvae may expire through dehydration. Ideally the temperature should be constant at around 18–23°C for temperate species of blowfly. It is recommended that a temperature datalogger is put into the incubator to obtain an accurate record of the temperature.

Blowfly eggs should be kept on moist tissue paper to maintain humidity because they are very susceptible to death by desiccation. As soon as larvae have hatched they should be placed into small pots (e.g. 50 ml disposable plastic cups) for rearing on a food substrate such as liver or dog food (see Section 8.4.1.3). Feeding larvae should be checked daily to ensure that they have enough food, and that they are not able to escape. Once the larvae are nearing the pupal stage, the pots should be placed into larger containers with sawdust or sterilised soil, into which they can disperse. The pupae will remain in their immobile state for a number of days, but care should be taken to ensure that the pots remain covered but still aerated (e.g. with gauze) to ensure that when the adult flies emerge they cannot escape. While some blowfly species (e.g. *Calliphora vicina*) will pupariate in a relatively dry environment such as sawdust, others are less tolerant of low humidities (e.g. *Lucilia caesar*) and will not pupariate unless the substrate is moist.

It is important to ensure that all rearing pots are clearly labelled with their original data, including case and sample number, and that different samples are not mixed. Insects being reared through to the adult stage should be checked on a daily basis, and a record of visit times and stage of the insect development on each occasion noted. It is especially important to note down the date/time when the adult flies emerge. Once emerged, the adults should be removed from the sample, so as not to confuse these adults with ones that emerge over the following days, killed by placing in a freezer for one or more hours, and then pinned and identified. Each pin should also be labelled with the appropriate information for that specimen, including sample number and time/date of adult emergence.

8.6.2   Insect identification

Identification of all specimens, both immature and adult, is the essential first stage in any investigation of insect evidence. It should be undertaken by a trained entomologist, using a binocular microscope and reference to published identification keys (Greenberg and Kunich, 2002; Smith, 1986; Szpila, 2010; Thyssen, 2010). It is crucial that all samples are correctly identified to ensure an accurate estimation of PMI_{min}, because different (even closely related) species develop at different rates (Richards, Crous and Villet, 2009). If morphological identifications are not possible then molecular biological methods can be used to identify all life stages (Stevens and Wall, 2001). These should be carried out by someone familiar with molecular techniques to ensure accurate DNA extraction, analysis and interpretation.

8.6.3 Insect measurement

The life-stage of larvae should be determined (i.e. 1st, 2nd, 3rd instar, feeding/post-feeding) and they should also be measured in length using an eyepiece graticule or computer-based measuring software. There are an increasing number of publications which provide information on development of blowfly species in terms of development stage and/or larval length (Table 8.1). Less commonly, weight is used as a measure of age, however this parameter is much more variable than length and is therefore not recommended.

8.6.4 Estimating scene temperatures

Insect development occurs at a rate that is proportional to temperature such that between the upper and lower thermal limits for development of any species, cool temperatures will result in a longer period of development while warm temperatures

Table 8.1 Publications that contain developmental data on different blowfly species (Diptera: Calliphoridae) based on three or more temperatures.

Species	References
Calliphora vicina	Reiter, 1984; Williams and Richardson, 1984; Greenberg, 1991; Davies and Ratcliffe, 1994; Anderson, 2000; Marchenko, 2001; Donovan *et al.*, 2006
Calliphora vomitoria	Greenberg and Tantawi, 1993; Davies and Ratcliffe, 1994
Chrysomya albiceps	Queiroz, 1996; Al-Misned, 2001; Grassberger *et al.*, 2003; Richards *et al.*, 2008
Chrysomya megacephala	Nishida, 1984; Richards and Villet, 2009
Cochliomyia macellaria	Melvin, 1934; Byrd and Butler, 1996
Lucilia cuprina	Melvin, 1934; Buei, 1959; O'Flynn, 1983; Dallwitz, 1984; Williams and Richardson, 1984
Lucilia sericata	Melvin, 1934; Ash and Greenberg, 1975; Wall *et al.*, 1992; Davies and Ratcliffe, 1994; Anderson, 2000; Grassberger and Reiter, 2001; Marchenko, 2001; Bourel *et al.*, 2003
Phormia regina	Melvin, 1934; Nishida, 1984; Byrd and Allen, 2001
Protophormia terraenovae	Greenberg and Tantawi, 1993; Grassberger and Reiter, 2002

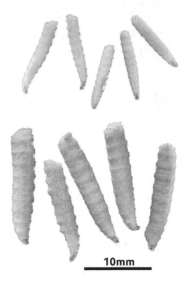

Figure 8.8 Blowfly larvae of the same age, 48 hrs old, which developed at 21°C (above) and 27°C (below).

will result in a shorter period of development (Figure 8.8). Therefore it is essential to estimate the temperatures at which the insects collected from the body were developing. Significant temperature variation can be recorded between different locations even only a short distance apart due to environmental features, for example open grassland, under a hedge, in a ditch. Because of this the forensic entomologist cannot rely on simply using temperature data from the nearest weather station. Likewise, uncertified weather data such as that available on some web sites should not be used. Instead, hourly temperatures should be recorded at the scene for a period of approximately 10 days using a digital temperature datalogger placed at the location where the body was found, ideally in a portable Stevenson screen if outdoors. A regression analysis should then be carried out of scene temperatures and those at a nearby weather station for the same period (Figure 8.9). The temperature at the scene before discovery of the body, usually back to the time of last confirmed live sighting of the victim, can then be estimated by applying the regression formula to the hourly data from the nearby weather station for that same period.

8.6.5 Estimating the age of insect evidence

It is important to always bear in mind that forensic entomology does not estimate the actual PMI or time-since-death but instead estimates the minimum (PMI_{min}). This is because what is actually determined from the age of the oldest insects is when they were first laid as eggs (for some species as larvae) on the body, which is not necessarily when death occurred. If the body was lying outdoors in summer

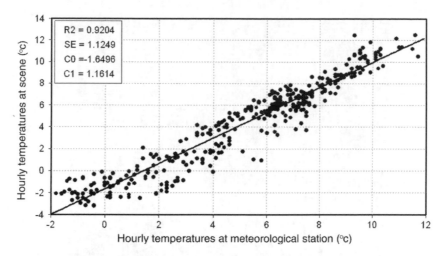

Figure 8.9 Linear regression of hourly temperature data of scene against local meteorological station, for a 16-day December period in the United Kingdom.

conditions then the primary colonisation could indeed occur within hours, or even minutes of death (Anderson, 2011). However, there can be many reasons for delayed colonisation if the body is concealed in some way, such as having been wrapped (Goff, 1992) or if it is first exposed during inclement weather (rain, cold) or in a season of low fly activity (e.g. winter or dry season). Even fires may not destroy insect evidence, although oviposition rates may be affected (Anderson, 2005). An indoor scene is an obvious example with potential for delayed colonisation and studies have shown that colonisation is indeed delayed, with fewer insects on indoor pig cadavers and an extended decomposition and insect colonisation period compared to outdoor bodies (Anderson, 2011; Reibe and Madea, 2010).

It is beyond the scope or objective of this chapter to go into detail regarding how insect age is determined from the available evidence, but more detailed information on this can be found in Byrd and Castner (2001, 2009). Estimation of PMI_{min} can be a relatively straightforward procedure by measuring the size or stage of the oldest insects and then checking databases of development (Table 8.1) to determine how long it would take them to reach that size or life stage at the temperatures estimated for the scene (Villet, Richards and Midgley, 2010). However, many highly variable factors need to be considered. One of these is the potential elevated temperature of a larval mass (Cianci and Sheldon, 1990; Rivers, Thompson and Brogan, 2011). The raised temperatures (Figure 8.10) would be expected to lead to more rapid development, but measurement of this is complicated because the larval mass temperature for the oldest specimens will not be a constant, increasing gradually from the 2nd instar stage, and the larval specimens will not necessarily be exposed to the highest temperatures for all of their development because these can approach the upper limits for survival. At present, although some compensation factors can be applied, there is no simple method to account for the effects of larval masses (Charabidze

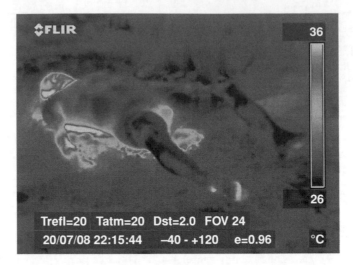

Figure 8.10   Infrared thermal image of human body showing increased temperatures at sites of larval masses, that is, on the head, the body–soil interface, and the anal-genital region. (To see a colour version of this figure, please see Plate 8.10.)

et al., 2011). However, in many cases a significant period of development within larval masses for the oldest insect stages is not observed and forensic entomology can still provide a very powerful tool for estimating PMI_{min}. Much basic and applied research is under way to further improve the manner in which insect evidence can be presented to meet the increasingly strict criteria required by courts since the *Daubert v. Merrell Dow Pharmaceuticals, Inc.* case of 1993 (Amendt *et al.*, 2010; Greenberg and Kunich, 2002; Tomberlin *et al.*, 2011).

8.7   Reporting and court appearance

Attendance in court is usually required only when the PMI is central to the case or in contention. However, the entomologist should be fully prepared to be called to court to give evidence, and it is therefore wise to have completed an Expert Witness course, and this might be a prerequisite for being considered for casework. If required to attend court, the entomologist should be suitably attired, arrive in good time and follow the instructions of the clerk of the court. Although a copy of the entomology report will usually be provided at court, it is advisable to take a copy that can be referred to in the witness stand.

The forensic entomologist will usually be asked to explain to the jury what forensic entomology is and how it can be used in criminal cases, and then to sum up their findings, as outlined in the report. Care should be taken to use language that will be understood easily by non-scientists, and to explain any unusual terms or processes. The entomologist will then be asked questions first by the prosecution and then the defence. Likely questions will focus on how the samples were collected, whether they met peer reviewed protocols, (e.g. Amendt *et al.*, 2007), why temperatures are so important to PMI estimation, the accuracy of forensic entomology estimates and what results were obtained.

8.8 Conclusion

Forensic entomology can make a highly effective contribution to criminal investigations, but in order for it to be of robust evidential value strict protocols should be followed with regard to collection and preservation of insect evidence, subsequent analysis and reporting. Ideally this should be conducted by an appropriately qualified forensic entomologist or under the guidance of such.

References

Adams, Z.J.O. and Hall, M.J.R. 2003. Methods used for the killing and preservation of blowfly larvae, and their effect on post-mortem larval length. *Forensic Science International* **138**: 50–61.

Al-Misned, F.A.M. 2001. Biological effects of cadmium on life cycle parameters of *Chrysomya albiceps* (Wiedemann) (Diptera: Calliphoridae). *Kuwait Journal of Science & Engineering* **28**: 179–188.

Amendt, J., Campobasso, C., Gaudry, E. *et al.* 2007. Best practice in forensic entomology – standards and guidelines. *International Journal of Legal Medicine* **121**: 90–104.

Amendt, J., Goff, M. L., Campobasso, C.P. and Grassberger, M. (eds) 2010. *Current Concepts in Forensic Entomology.* Springer, London.

Anderson, G.S. 1999. Wildlife forensic entomology: determining time of death in two illegally killed black bear cubs. *Journal of Forensic Sciences* **44**: 856–859.

Anderson, G.S. 2000. Minimum and maximum development rates of some forensically important Calliphoridae (Diptera). *Journal of Forensic Sciences* **45**: 824–832.

Anderson, G.S. 2005. Effects of arson on forensic entomology evidence. *Canadian Society of Forensic Science* **38**: 49–67.

Anderson, G.S. 2011. Comparison of decomposition rates and faunal colonization of carrion in indoor and outdoor environments. *Journal of Forensic Sciences* **56**: 136–142.

Anderson, G.S. and Huitson, N.R. 2004. Myiasis in pet animals: the potential of forensic entomology for determining duration of possible neglect. *Canadian Veterinary Journal* **45**: 993–998.

Anderson, G.S. and VanLaerhoven, S.L. 1996. Initial studies on insect succession on carrion in Southwestern British Columbia. *Journal of Forensic Sciences* **41**: 617–625.

Ash, N. and Greenberg, B. 1975. Developmental temperature responses of the sibling species *Phaenicia sericata* and *Phaenicia pallescens. Annals of the Entomological Society of America* **68**: 197–200.

Benecke, M. 2004. Arthropods and corpses. In M. Tsokos (ed.) *Forensic Pathology Reviews.* Humana Press Inc., Totowa, NJ, pp. 207–240.

Benecke, M. and Lessig, R. 2001. Child neglect and forensic entomology. *Forensic Science International* **120**: 155–159.

Bourel, B., Callet, B., Hédouin, V. and Gosset, D. 2003. Flies eggs: a new method for the estimation of short-term post-mortem interval? *Forensic Science International* **135**: 27–34.

Buei, V.K. 1959. The life-history of the sheep blowfly, *Lucilia cuprina* Wiedemann. Ecological studies of the flies of medical importance. *Botyu-Kagaku* **24**: 115–118.

Byrd, J.H. and Allen, J.C. 2001. The development of the black blow fly, *Phormia regina* (Meigen). *Forensic Science International* **120**: 79–88.

Byrd, J.H. and Butler, J.F. 1996. Effects of temperature on *Cochliomyia macellaria* (Diptera: Calliphoridae) development. *Journal of Medical Entomology* **33**: 901–905.

Byrd, J.H. and Castner, J.L. 2001. *Forensic Entomology: The Utility of Arthropods in Legal Investigations*. CRC Press, Boca Raton, FL.

Byrd, J.H. and Castner, J.L. 2009. *Forensic Entomology: The Utility of Arthropods in Legal Investigations*, 2nd edn. CRC Press, Boca Raton, FL.

Catts, E.P. and Haskell, N.H. 1990. *Entomology and Death: A Procedural Guide*. Joyce's Print Shop, Clemson, SC.

Charabidze, D., Bourel, B. and Gosset, D. 2011. Larval-mass effect: characterisation of heat emission by necrophageous blowflies (Diptera: Calliphoridae) larval aggregates. *Forensic Science International* **211**: 61–66.

Cianci, T.J. and Sheldon, J.K. 1990. Endothermic generation by blow fly larvae *Phormia regina* developing in pig carcasses. *Bulletin of the Society of Vector Ecology* **15**: 33–40.

Dallwitz, R. 1984. The influence of constant and fluctuating temperatures on development rate and survival of pupae of the Australian sheep blowfly *Lucilia sericata*. *Entomologia Experimentalis et Applicata* **36**: 89–95.

Davies, L. and Ratcliffe, G.G. 1994. Developmental rates of some pre-adult stages in blowflies with reference to low temperatures. *Medical and Veterinary Entomology* **8**: 245–254.

de Carvalho, L.M.L. 2010. Toxicology and forensic entomology. In J. Amendt, C.P. Campobasso, L.M. Goff and M. Grassberger (eds) *Current Concepts in Forensic Entomology*. Springer, London, pp. 163–178.

Disney, R.H.L. 1994. *Scuttle flies: the Phoridae*. Chapman and Hall, London.

Donovan, S.E., Hall, M.J.R., Turner, B.D. and Moncrieff, C.B. 2006. Larval growth rates of the blowfly, *Calliphora vicina*, over a range of temperatures. *Medical and Veterinary Entomology* **20**: 1–9.

Drijfhout, F.P. 2010. Cuticular hydrocarbons: a new tool in forensic entomology? In J. Amendt, C.P. Campobasso, L.M. Goff and M. Grassberger (eds) *Current Concepts in Forensic Entomology*. Springer, London, pp. 179–203.

Easton, A.M. and Smith, K.G.V. 1970. The entomology of the cadaver. *Medical Science Law* **10**: 208–215.

Erzinçlioğlu, Z. 1996. *Blowflies*. Naturalists' Handbooks 23. The Richmond Publishing Co. Ltd., Slough.

Erzinçlioğlu, Z. 2000. *Maggots, Murder and Men: Memories and Reflections of a Forensic Entomologist*. Harley Books, Colchester.

Gaudry E. 2010. The insects colonisation of buried remains. In J. Amendt, C.P. Campobasso, L.M. Goff and M. Grassberger (eds) *Current Concepts in Forensic Entomology*. Springer, London, pp. 273–311.

Gennard, D.E. 2007. *Forensic Entomology: An Introduction*. John Wiley & Sons, Ltd, Chichester.

Goff, M.L. 1992. Problems in estimation of postmortem interval resulting from wrapping of the corpse: a case study from Hawaii. *Journal of Agricultural Entomology* **9**: 237–243.

Goff, M.L. 2000. *A Fly for the Prosecution – How Insect Evidence Helps Solve Crimes*. Harvard University Press, Cambridge, MA.

Grassberger, M. and Reiter, C. 2001. Effect of temperature on *Lucilia sericata* (Diptera: Calliphoridae) development with special reference to the isomegalen- and isomorphen-diagram. *Forensic Science International* **120**: 32–36.

Grassberger, M. and Reiter, C. 2002. Effect of temperature on development of the forensically important holarctic blow fly *Protophormia terraenovae* (Robineau-Desvoidy) (Diptera: Calliphoridae). *Forensic Science International* **28**: 177–182.

Grassberger, M., Friedrich, M. and Reiter, C. 2003. The blowfly *Chrysomya albiceps* (Wiedemann) (Diptera: Calliphoridae) as a new forensic indicator in central Europe. *International Journal of Legal Medicine* **117**: 75–81.

Greenberg, B. 1991. Flies as forensic indicators. *Journal of Medical Entomology* **28**: 565–577.

Greenberg, B. and Kunich, J.C. 2002. *Entomology and the Law: Flies as Forensic Indicators*. Cambridge University Press, Cambridge.

Greenberg, B. and Tantawi, T.I. 1993. Different developmental strategies in two boreal blow flies (Diptera: Calliphoridae). *Journal of Medical Entomology* **30**: 481–484.

Gunn, A. and Bird, J. 2011. The ability of the blowflies *Calliphora vomitoria* (Linnaeus), *Calliphora vicina* (Rob-Desvoidy) and *Lucilia sericata* (Meigen) (Diptera: Calliphoridae) and the muscid flies *Muscina stabulans* (Fallén) and *Muscina prolapsa* (Harris) (Diptera: Muscidae) to colonise buried remains. *Forensic Science International* **207**: 198–204.

Hall, M.J.R. and Smith, K.G.V. 1993. Diptera causing myiasis in man. In R.P. Lane and R.W. Crosskey (eds) *Medical Insects and Arachnids*. Chapman and Hall, London, pp. 429–469.

Hall, M.J.R. and Wall, R. 1995. Myiasis of humans and domestic animals. *Advances in Parasitology* **35**: 257–334.

Hall, M.J.R., Brown, T., Jones, P. and Clark, D. 2008. Forensic sciences. In M. Cox, A. Flavel, I. Hanson, J. Laver and R. Wessling (eds) *The Scientific Investigation of Mass Graves: Towards Protocols and Standard Operating Procedures*. Cambridge University Press, Cambridge, pp. 463–497.

Hall, R.D. 1990. Medicocriminal entomology. In E.P. Catts and N.H. Haskell (eds) *Entomology and Death: A Procedural Guide*. Joyce's Print Shop, Clemson, SC.

Hall, R.D. 2001. Introduction: Perceptions and status of forensic entomology. In J.H. Byrd and J.L. Castner (eds) *Forensic Entomology: The Utility of Arthropods in Legal Investigations*. CRC Press, Boca Raton, FL, pp. 1–15.

Hart, A.J., Whitaker, A.P. and Hall, M.J.R. 2008. The use of forensic entomology in criminal investigations: how it can be of benefit to SIOs. *The Journal of Homicide and Major Incident Investigation* **4**: 37–47.

Haskell, N.H. and Williams, R.E. (eds) 2008. *Entomology and Death: A Procedural Guide*. Joyce's Print Shop, Clemson, SC.

Henssge, C., Madea, B. and Gallenkemper, E. 1988. Death time estimation in case work. II. Integration of different methods. *Forensic Science International* **39**: 77–87.

Hira, P.R., Assad, R., Oshaka, G. *et al.* 2004. Myiasis in Kuwait: nosocomial infections caused by *Lucilia* and *Megaselia* species. *American Journal of Tropical Medicine and Hygiene* **70**: 386–389.

Johl, H.K. and Anderson, G.S. 1996. Effects of refrigeration on development of the blow fly, *Calliphora vicina* (Diptera: Calliphoridae) and their relationship to time of death. *Journal of the Entomological Society of British Columbia* **93**: 93–98.

Kumara, T.K., Abu Hassan, A., Che Salmah, M.R and Bhupinder, S. 2009. The infestation of *Dermestes ater* (De Geer) on a human corpse in Malaysia. *Tropical Biomedicine* **26**: 73–79.

Lord, W.D. 1990. Case histories of the use of insects in investigations. In E.P. Catts and N.H. Haskell (eds) *Entomology and Death: A Procedural Guide*. Joyce's Print Shop, Clemson, SC, pp. 9–37.

Lord, W.D. and Stevenson, J.R. 1986. *American Registered Professional Entomologists*. Chesapeake Chapter, Washington DC.

Marchenko, M.I. 2001. Medicolegal relevance of cadaver entomofauna for the determination of the time of death. *Forensic Science International* **120**: 89–109.

Matuszewski, S., Bajerlein, D., Konwerski, S. and Szpila, K. 2011. Insect succession and carrion decomposition in selected forests of Central Europe. Part 3: Succession of carrion fauna. *Forensic Science International* **207**: 150–163.

Mégnin, P. 1894. *La Faune des Cadavres*. Encyclopédie Scientifique des Aide-Mémoire. G. Masson and Gauthier-Villars et Fils, Paris.

Melvin, R. 1934. Incubation period of eggs of certain muscoid flies at different constant temperatures. *Annals of the Entomological Society of America* **27**: 406–410.

Midgley, J.M., Richards, C.S. and Villet, M.H. 2010. The utility of Coleoptera in forensic investigations. In J. Amendt, C.P. Campobasso, L.M. Goff and M. Grassberger (eds) *Current Concepts in Forensic Entomology*. Springer, London, pp. 57–68.

Nishida, K. 1984. Experimental studies on the estimation of postmortem intervals by means of fly larvae infesting human cadavers. *Japanese Journal of Forensic Medicine* **38**: 24–41.

O'Flynn, M.A. 1983. The succession and rate of development of blowflies in carrion in southern Queensland and the application of these data to forensic entomology. *Journal of the Australian Entomological Society* **22**: 137–148.

Payne, J.A., King, E.W. and Beinhart, G. 1968. Arthropod succession and decomposition of buried pigs. *Nature* **219**: 1180–1181.

Queiroz, M.M.C. 1996. Temperature requirements of *Chrysomya albiceps* (Wiedemann, 1819) (Diptera: Calliphoridae) under laboratory conditions. *Memórias Do Instituto Oswaldo Cruz* **91**: 1–6.

Reibe, S. and Madea, B. 2010. How promptly do blowflies colonise fresh carcasses? A study comparing indoor with outdoor locations. *Forensic Science International* **195**: 52–57.

Reiter, C. 1984. Zum Wachstumsverhalten der Maden der blauen Schmeißfliege *Calliphora vicina*. *Zeitschrift für Rechtsmedizin* **91**: 295–308.

Richards, C.S. and Villet, M.H. 2009. Data quality in thermal summation models of development of forensically important blowflies. *Medical and Veterinary Entomology* **23**: 269–276.

Richards, C.S., Crous, K.L. and Villet, M.H. 2009. Models of development for blowfly sister species *Chrysomya chloropyga* and *Chrysomya putoria*. *Medical and Veterinary Entomology* **23**: 56–61.

Richards, C.S., Paterson, I.H. and Villet, M.H. 2008. Estimating the age of immature *Chrysomya albiceps* (Diptera: Calliphoridae), correcting for temperature and geographic latitude. *International Journal of Legal Medicine* **122**: 401–408.

Rivers, D.B., Thompson, C. and Brogan, R. 2011. Physiological trade-offs of forming maggot masses by necrophagous flies on vertebrate carrion. *Bulletin of Entomological Research* **101**: 599–611.

Roeterdink, E.M., Dadour, I.R. and Watling, R.J. 2004. Extraction of gunshot residues from the larvae of the forensically important blowfly *Calliphora dubia* (Macquart) (Diptera: Calliphoridae). *International Journal of Legal Medicine* **118**: 63–70.

Samuel, W.M. 1988. The use of age classes of winter ticks on moose to determine time of death. *Canadian Society of Forensic Science Journal* **21**: 54–59.

Singh, D. and Greenberg, B. 1994. Survival after submergence in the pupae of five species of blow flies (Diptera: Calliphoridae). *Journal of Medical Entomology* **31**: 757–759.

Smith, K.G.V. 1986. *A Manual of Forensic Entomology*. British Museum (Natural History) and Cornell University Press, Ithaca.

Stevens, J. and Wall, R. 2001. Genetic relationships between blowflies (Calliphoridae) of forensic importance. *Forensic Science International* **120**: 116–123.

Swift, B. 2010. Methods of time since death estimation within the early post-mortem interval. *The Journal of Homicide and Major Incident Investigation* **6**: 97–112.

Szpila, K. 2010. Key for the identification of third instars of European blowflies (Diptera; Calliphoridae) of forensic importance. In J. Amendt, C.P. Campobasso, L.M. Goff and M. Grassberger (eds) *Current Concepts in Forensic Entomology*. Springer, London, pp. 43–56.

Szpila, K., Voss J.G. and Pape, T. 2010. A new dipteran forensic indicator in buried bodies. *Medical and Veterinary Entomology* **24**: 278–283.

Tantawi, T.I. and Greenberg, B. 1993. The effects of killing and preservation solutions on estimates of larval age in forensic cases. *Journal of Forensic Sciences* **38**: 702–707.

Thyssen, P.J. 2010. Keys for identification of immature insects. In J. Amendt, C.P. Campobasso, L.M. Goff and M. Grassberger (eds) *Current Concepts in Forensic Entomology*. Springer, London, pp. 25–42.

Tomberlin, J.K., Mohr, R., Benbow, M.E. *et al.* 2011. A roadmap for bridging basic and applied research in forensic entomology. *Annual Review of Entomology* **56**: 401–421.

Villet, M.H., Richards, C.S. and Midgley, J.M. 2010. Contemporary precision, bias and accuracy of minimum post-mortem intervals estimated using development of carrion-feeding insects. In J. Amendt, C.P. Campobasso, L.M. Goff and M. Grassberger (eds) *Current Concepts in Forensic Entomology*. Springer, London, pp. 109–137.

Wall, R., French, N. and Morgan, K.L. 1992. Effects of temperature on the development and abundance of the sheep blowfly *Lucilia sericata* (Diptera: Calliphoridae). *Bulletin of Entomological Research* **82**: 125–131.

Wells J.D., Introna F. Jr, Di Vella, G. *et al.* 2001. Human and insect mitochondrial DNA analysis from maggots. *Journal of Forensic Science* **46**: 685–687.

Wells, J.D. and King, J. 2001. Incidence of precocious egg development in flies of forensic importance (Calliphoridae). *Pan-Pacific Entomologist* **77**: 235–239.

Wells, J.D. and Lamotte, L.R. 2001. Estimating the postmortem interval. In J.H. Byrd and J.L. Castner (eds) *Forensic Entomology: The Utility of Arthropods in Legal Investigations*. CRC Press, Boca Raton, FL, pp. 263–285.

Williams, H. and Richardson, A.M.M. 1984. Growth energetics in relation to temperature for larvae of four species of necrophagous flies (Diptera: Calliphoridae). *Australian Journal of Ecology* **9**: 141–152.

Appendix 8.1   Entomological collection scene sheet (based on Amendt *et al.*, 2007).

Collected by:_____Date_____Case No_____

Entomological Collection Scene Sheet

Client Name_____

Contact Name_____

Client Address_____

_____

_____

Telephone Number_____

Police Force (if not client)_____

Time of arrival:_____ Time of departure:_____

Scene of Recovery / Mortuary (delete as applicable)

Persons Present

Name	Job Title	Company

Address of Scene/ Mortuary   _____

_____

_____

_____

_____

_____

Approved by: Name .... Signature .... Date ....

Appendix 8.1 (*Continued*)

Collected by:_____Date_____Case No_____

<u>**Specifications of deceased (Known / Estimate)**</u>

Age _____Gender _____Height_____ Weight _____

Position (tick more than one if appropriate):

Indoor ☐   Outdoor ☐   Aquatic ☐   Buried ☐ (estimated depth:_____)

Concealed ☐   Hanging ☐ (In contact with ground) Yes / No

Clothing:
Fully clothed ☐   Partial ☐ (record partial clothing on body sketch)   Naked ☐

Covering:
Fully covered ☐   Partial ☐   (record partial cover on body sketch)

Body covered with:_____

General state of decomposition:

Fresh ☐   bloated ☐   active decay ☐   advanced decay ☐   dry/skeletal ☐
(if more than one decomposition state, record position on body sketch)

Mark the positions and provide details for evidence of scavenging or trauma on body sketch

<u>**Scene of recovery (tick more than one box where appropriate)**</u>

Urban ☐   Rural ☐

Outdoor:

Vegetation:

Woodland/Forest ☐   Grassland ☐   Heath ☐   Marshland ☐   Agricultural ☐

Other _____

Substrate:

Clay ☐   Sand ☐   Stony ☐   Man-made ☐ (define:_____)

Other_____

Exposure: Sun ☐   Shade ☐   Partial shade ☐

Indoor:

Building zone: Residential ☐   Commercial ☐   Industrial ☐   Agricultural ☐

Building type: Apartment/Flat ☐   House ☐   Garage/Storage ☐   Stable/Barn ☐

Other: _____

Approved by: Name .... Signature .... Date ....

Appendix 8.1   *(Continued)*

Collected by:_____Date_____Case No_____

Room: Kitchen   ☐   Bedroom ☐   Bathroom ☐   Living Room   ☐

Dining room   ☐   Passage/Hallway/Entrance Hall ☐   Staircase   ☐

Store room   ☐   Study   ☐   Loft   ☐   Cellar   ☐

Other:_____

Record details of dispersing insect evidence on Sampling Sheet

Floor level: _____

*Floor type (carpet, wood, concrete, etc.):*_____

Heated: ☐   *Thermostat setting:* _____

Insect access: Windows – Open ☐   Closed ☐   Ajar ☐

                  Doors   – Open ☐   Closed ☐   Ajar ☐

Miscellaneous (e.g. car):_____

_____

_____

_____

Temperatures

Ambient 1 (2 m above ground): _____

*Ambient 2 (5 cm above ground):*_____

Body surface: _____

(If present) larval mass 1*:_____   larval mass 4*:_____
              larval mass 2*:_____   larval mass 5*:_____
              larval mass 3*:_____   larval mass 6*:_____

* please mark the positions on body sketch

*Interface between body and ground:*_____

Soil(at a depth of about 20 cm): _____

Water: _____

Record air temperature at scene of recovery for 5–10 days after discovery of body

Datalogger left at scene? **Y / N**   Serial no._____ Stevenson Screen? **Y / N**

Datalogger with live samples? **Y / N**   Serial no._____

Approved by: Name .... Signature .... Date ....

Appendix 8.1 (*Continued*)

Collected by:_____ Date_____ Case No_____

Key

Shade for partial clothing/cover ▨

F	fresh	EM_1, EM_2	egg masses
B	bloated	LM_1, LM_2	larval masses
AC	active decay	W	wandering larvae
AD	advanced decay	P	pupae
D	dry/skeletal	EP	empty pupal cases
SC	scavenging	F	flies
T	trauma sites	B	beetles

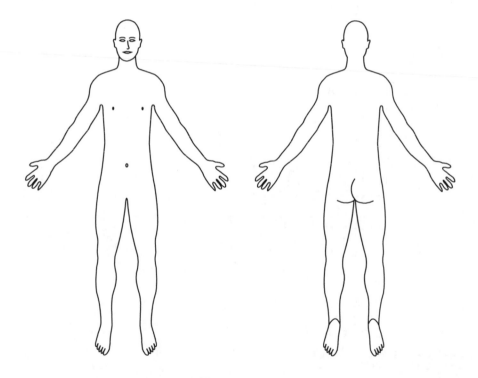

Approved by: Name .... Signature .... Date ....

Appendix 8.1   (*Continued*)

Collected by:_____Date_____Case No_____

Sampling Sheet

E = Eggs	L = Feeding Larvae*
W = Wandering larvae**	P = Pupae
EP = Empty pupal cases	F = Flies
B = Beetles	

Sample N°	Approx. number	Type	Preserved (P) / Alive (A)	Location on body/scene ^
1		E ☐ L ☐ W ☐ P ☐ EP ☐ F ☐ B ☐		
2		E ☐ L ☐ W ☐ P ☐ EP ☐ F ☐ B ☐		
3		E ☐ L ☐ W ☐ P ☐ EP ☐ F ☐ B ☐		
4		E ☐ L ☐ W ☐ P ☐ EP ☐ F ☐ B ☐		
5		E ☐ L ☐ W ☐ P ☐ EP ☐ F ☐ B ☐		
6		E ☐ L ☐ W ☐ P ☐ EP ☐ F ☐ B ☐		
7		E ☐ L ☐ W ☐ P ☐ EP ☐ F ☐ B ☐		
8		E ☐ L ☐ W ☐ P ☐ EP ☐ F ☐ B ☐		
9		E ☐ L ☐ W ☐ P ☐ EP ☐ F ☐ B ☐		
10		E ☐ L ☐ W ☐ P ☐ EP ☐ F ☐ B ☐		
11		E ☐ L ☐ W ☐ P ☐ EP ☐ F ☐ B ☐		
12		E ☐ L ☐ W ☐ P ☐ EP ☐ F ☐ B ☐		
13		E ☐ L ☐ W ☐ P ☐ EP ☐ F ☐ B ☐		
14		E ☐ L ☐ W ☐ P ☐ EP ☐ F ☐ B ☐		
15		E ☐ L ☐ W ☐ P ☐ EP ☐ F ☐ B ☐		
16		E ☐ L ☐ W ☐ P ☐ EP ☐ F ☐ B ☐		
17		E ☐ L ☐ W ☐ P ☐ EP ☐ F ☐ B ☐		
18		E ☐ L ☐ W ☐ P ☐ EP ☐ F ☐ B ☐		

Preserved = killed in boiling water and preserved in 80% ethanol
Alive = keep them alive e.g. for rearing
* Larvae feeding on the body
** Larvae no longer feeding on the body, i.e. dispersing from the body, or hiding in clothes, in soil, under furniture and so forth
^ mark the positions on the body sketch

Approved by: Name ………………………………. Signature ……………………………………. Date …………………….

9

Diatoms and forensic science

Eileen J. Cox
Natural History Museum, London, UK

9.1 Introduction

9.1.1 What are diatoms?

Diatoms are an extremely species-rich (<200 000 species) (Mann and Droop, 1996), widely distributed group of microalgae (photosynthetic microscopic organisms), occurring in almost all illuminated aquatic environments, both freshwater and marine, from the equator to the poles (Figure 9.1). Cells are typically less than 100 µm maximum dimension (although a small number of species can be larger), and are distinguished by the possession of variously structured, essentially bipartite, siliceous cell walls (frustules), the construction of which is best seen using scanning electron microscopy (Figure 9.2) (Round, Crawford and Mann, 1990). Diatoms essentially function as single cells but can form colonies or filaments, particularly if they live in the plankton. Other species attach to submerged surfaces, or are actively motile over sediments. Because of the resistant nature of silica, diatoms are readily preserved in sediments, especially in lakes, which has led to their extensive use in palaeolimnology (Battarbee *et al.*, 1984). Under particular ecological circumstances, where nutrient-rich water has resulted in high diatom production, they can also form extensive geological deposits, diatomites (Harwood, 2010).

Whilst being widely distributed as a group, individual diatom species respond characteristically to environmental conditions, such that different habitats are typically colonised by different species, and there may also be seasonal variation in the growth of particular species (Reynolds, 2006; Round, 1981; Stevenson, Bothwell and Lowe, 1996). As a result, diatom assemblages will not only differ between water bodies with differing physical and chemical characteristics, but can also show variation between habitats and seasons within those water bodies (Cox, 1988, 1990a,b,c). They are therefore extensively used as indicators of ecological conditions, both contemporary and historical (Smol and Stoermer, 2010), and

Forensic Ecology Handbook: From Crime Scene to Court, First Edition.
Edited by Nicholas Márquez-Grant and Julie Roberts.
© 2012 John Wiley & Sons, Ltd. Published 2012 by John Wiley & Sons, Ltd.

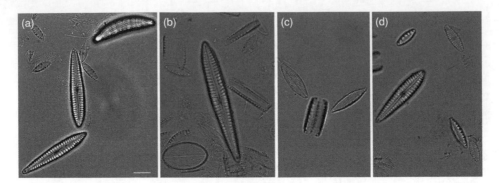

Figure 9.1 Light micrographs of cleaned diatoms valves from freshwater, showing specimens of *Gomphonema* (a,b,d), *Rhopalodia* (a), *Cocconeis* (b), *Nitzschia* (b,c – girdle view), and *Navicula* (c,d). Scale bar = 10 μm.

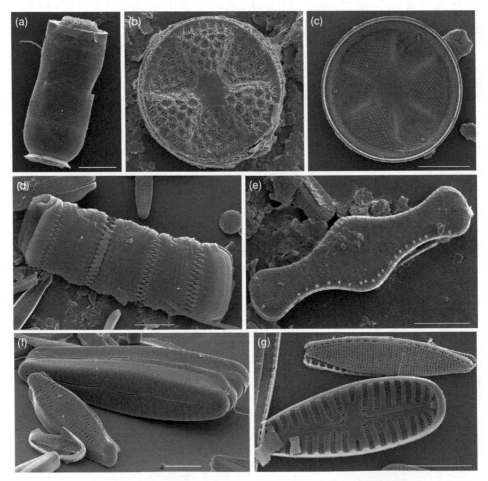

Figure 9.2 Scanning electron micrographs showing contrasting construction of different diatom genera. *Melosira* (a); *Actinoptychus* exterior (b); *Actinoptychus* interior (c); *Staurosira* (d); *Tabellaria* (e); *Gomphonema* exterior (f); *Gomphonema* interior and *Nitzschia* exterior (g). Scale bars = 10 μm (a,b,c) and 5 μm (d,e,f,g).

qualitative predictions can be made by diatom analysts about the type of locality supporting diatom assemblages of unknown provenance, as shown by a quality assurance exercise performed by the Forensic Science Service in the United Kingdom (Peabody and Cameron, 2010).

9.1.1.1 Diatom species and identification

Diatom species have been defined and recognised on the basis of the features of their silica cell walls, with particular emphasis on shape, symmetry, arrangement of pores and other features (Cox, 2011). Scanning electron microscopy has revealed much more fine-structural variation, but for routine purposes most diatom samples are analysed using light microscopy, under oil immersion. Although it is possible to identify many diatoms from fresh (live) material, using protoplast features such as chloroplast shape, number and position (Cox, 1996), most work has relied on the cell walls after cell contents have been removed by oxidation. Once 'cleaned' in this way, permanent slides can be made and retained for examination at any time.

Although molecular approaches are modifying our understanding of the evolutionary relationships of diatoms (Theriot *et al.*, 2009, 2010), the traditional classification based on valve shape, symmetry and valve patterning allows many genera to be readily identified, while more subtle variations in size, outline, pore arrangement and density discriminate between species. Thus, for identification purposes it is useful to recognise three main groups of diatoms based on the shape and symmetry of their valves: centric, araphid and raphid pennates. Centric diatoms have circular or multi-angular valves, with a radiating arrangement of pores, whereas pennate diatoms have a long axis of symmetry, with more or less transversely arranged rows of pores, perpendicular to the long axis. Raphid and araphid diatoms are recognised respectively on the presence or absence of a raphe system, that is, paired slits through the valve that facilitate movement over surfaces. A number of keys to common diatom genera and species have been published (Barber and Haworth, 1981; Kelly, 2000; Sonnemann *et al.*, 2000; Taylor, Harding and Archibald, 2007), or are available online (*A taxonomic key to the diatoms of South African Rivers*), as software designed for water quality monitoring, for example OMNIDIA, or CD (*Common freshwater diatoms of Britain and Ireland*). Identification to species relies on more specialist floras, for example Krammer and Lange-Bertalot (1986, 1988, 1991a,b), accounts of floras of particular areas, in series such as *Iconographia Diatomologica* or *Diatoms of Europe*, or in taxonomic papers published in scientific journals, such as *Diatom Research* and more general phycological journals such as the *European Journal of Phycology* and *Journal of Phycology*.

9.1.2 Why are diatoms useful in criminal investigation?

The ubiquity and site specificity of diatoms, combined with their small size and thus invisibility to the naked eye, renders them extremely useful as trace evidence, while their occurrence in water means that they can be used in assessments of drowning as a possible cause of death (Horton, 2007; Horton, Boreham and Hillier, 2006; Keiper and Casamatta, 2001; Peabody and Cameron, 2010). In addition, because under most circumstances their siliceous cell walls are not susceptible to deterioration, the evidence that they provide will persist longer than for some other biological material. It may also be possible to utilise information about growth rates of diatoms to infer length of exposure of material in water or damp environments (Casamatta and Verb, 2000; Keiper and Casamatta, 2001; Zimmerman and Wallace, 2008).

9.2 Applications

In a forensic context diatoms are probably most often used in tests for drowning. Drowning occurs when water enters the lungs and then, by rupturing the alveoli, the bloodstream, whence it can penetrate major organs and muscles, as can particles suspended in the drowning water (Piette and De Letter, 2006). Since diatoms are frequently found in natural fresh and marine waters, they are likely to be taken up during drowning and can be transported in the bloodstream. This is most likely when they are abundant in the water column, for example during spring and autumn freshwater blooms, when they may penetrate to the bone marrow (Pollanen, Cheung and Chaisson, 1997). On the other hand, diatoms are rarely found in domestic water supplies, at least in the United Kingdom (Peabody, 1999), although where they are found in water supplies, they can again be used to assist in the diagnosis of drowning (Pollanen, 1998). However, diatoms can be deposited in human organs before death (Peabody and Burgess, 1984) and the absence of diatoms does not necessarily exclude the possibility of drowning (Piette and De Letter, 2006; Pollanen et al., 1997).

Diatoms can also be used as trace evidence, where material from the scene of a crime has been deposited on clothing or shoes. This can be a result of the individual going through water containing diatoms (Peabody and Cameron, 2010), or from sediment or soil (Cameron, 2004; Siver, Lord and McCarthy, 1994), or from picking up material that contains diatoms or diatomite (diatomaceous earth) (Morgan and Bull, 2007; Peabody, 1999). Diatomite was often used as a fire-retardant in old safes and if such safes were broken open, diatomaceous earth would escape as a fine white powder and be deposited on clothing. Since an individual is unlikely to encounter diatomaceous earth by chance, such association was good evidence of presence at the scene of the crime (Peabody and Cameron, 2010). The presence of diatoms on clothing has similarly been used to link individuals to crime scenes (Peabody and Cameron, 2010); the match between the specimens on the clothing and in the natural environment indicating the likelihood of their provenance. It must, however, be noted that the quantity of diatoms in the environment, the nature of the clothing and duration of immersion, will all affect the extent to which diatoms are transferred to clothing.

Using diatoms to indicate length of exposure at a site, either to estimate time of death or provenance of an item is a more recent development (Casmatta and Verb, 2000; Zimmerman and Wallace, 2008) that requires knowledge of algal growth rates and prevailing environmental conditions. However, in the same way that entomological data can allow time of death to be estimated, extent of algal/diatom colonisation may provide useful information if there is sufficient empirical data on their growth patterns (Keiper and Casamatta, 2001).

Diatomite is used extensively for filtration in the brewing industry (Moores, 2008), in the production of fruit juice, sugar and edible oil, and also for filtering water for drinking supplies and public baths. It has been widely used as an abrasive in toothpaste and sink cleaners, as a filler in a variety of products, including paper, paint and cosmetics, as a thermal insulator and an absorbent (Harwood, 2010). It is also used as a mechanical insecticide and in cat litter. Although most diatomite is mined in the United States, other supplies come from China, Denmark, France, Japan and Mexico. If a product contains diatomite from a particular location, its characteristic diatom composition (determined by light microscopy) may be a useful indicator of provenance. The presence of unusual rare specimens of diatoms in nature can sometimes be traced back to the historical use of diatomite in the area (Clarke, 1991).

9.3   Pre-scene attendance

In preparing to attend a crime scene to sample diatoms, it is important to determine what type of sample or samples should be taken, and to bear in mind that diatom assemblages change with time. Thus, because the diatom assemblage in the water column will alter over time, it is unlikely that assemblages can be matched precisely when more than a few days or a week have elapsed between estimated time of crime and the investigation, particularly under warmer conditions. On the other hand, even allowing for seasonal variation, there will be consistent differences between diatom floras from different locations and habitats (Round, 1981), so it may still be useful to take environmental samples.

9.4   Scene attendance and sampling

Any suitably trained individual can take samples for diatom analysis, bearing in mind the need to avoid potential cross-contamination. Clear and careful labelling of all samples is essential (location, nature of sample, date) and, if they do not need to be fixed, samples should be kept cool and in the dark for transportation. It is useful to take samples both from the water column (near the surface), and from sediments and stone scrapings (see below), keeping the different types of sample separate. This will ensure that the full range of diatoms at the site is collected, together with information on their location.

Since they occur in illuminated, damp or aquatic habitats, diatoms can be sampled both from the water column, and from submerged or moist surfaces. Water samples can be taken using sterile bottles, while sediment samples can be taken using a spatula or short surface corer, and stones can be sampled by scraping or brushing. Because it is important to ensure that there is no cross-contamination, all sampling tools and containers should be clean and ideally sterile. Waterproof pens are required for labelling, and if there is likely to be a significant delay in processing, it may be necessary to have a suitable fixative such as formalin or alcohol to preserve the sample. While it is probably advisable to take litre water samples, which can then be concentrated, sediment samples need only be of a few cubic centimetres in volume, as this will provide sufficient diatoms for analysis.

Where it is suspected that diatom-containing substances have been transferred from the crime scene to the perpetrator, samples at the scene should be taken in small vials or bags, as for any other trace evidence, again ensuring that cross-contamination does not occur.

In the mortuary, the forensic pathologist will usually submit a sample of lung and another organ, such as kidney or liver, although it will also depend on the state of decomposition and any peri-mortem damage inflicted on those organs.

9.5 Preparation and treatment of samples in the laboratory

With the exception of samples of diatomite, which contain little organic material, most diatom-containing samples must be treated with oxidising agents to remove organics before they can be examined under the light microscope. For environmental samples in which there are abundant diatoms, it may be sufficient to treat the samples with inorganic acid or hydrogen peroxide, followed by washing, but for tissue samples it has been suggested that this is preceded by ashing in a muffle furnace to cope with larger volumes of organic material (Peabody, 1999; Peabody and Cameron, 2010). However, regardless of the precise preparation techniques employed, it is essential that all steps are taken to avoid any possible cross-contamination, using new, unused, clean laboratory ware and membrane-filtered reagents (Peabody and Cameron, 2010). It is also important to follow proper safety procedures at all times, particularly bearing potential health hazards in mind when dealing with body organs of unknown history.

For tissue samples therefore the procedure is as follows:

1. Weigh out 100 g sample of tissue into an evaporating dish.

2. Transfer to a muffle oven and heat for 3–5 h at 250°C.

3. Ash overnight at 550°C and allow to cool.

4. Dissolve resulting white ash in concentrated hydrochloric acid.

5. Wash several times in distilled water, centrifuging between washes.

6. If any organic matter remains, treat with concentrated nitric or sulphuric acid as per normal diatom preparation.

7. Wash well as before.

8. Dry aliquots of the final suspension onto cover slips and mount in high refractive index mountant, such as Naphrax, following manufacturer's instructions for curing.

Environmental samples should be transferred to small pyrex beakers in a fume cupboard, adding concentrated nitric or sulphuric acid and heating gently until the volume is reduced by at least half and the overlying liquid is clear. As above, wash several times with distilled water. Aliquots of the clean diatom suspension can then be dried onto cover slips and mounted as above. For marine samples it is advisable to wash the samples with distilled water before treating with acid. If samples are likely to contain carbonates, either pre-treat with hydrochloric acid (which will cause effervescence) and wash well before using sulphuric acid, or use only nitric acid to avoid the creation of insoluble precipitates.

9.6 Analysis of samples

Once permanent slides of samples have been prepared, these can be examined under the light microscope for diatoms or diatom fragments. Species identifications are best made under $\times 100$ objectives and oil immersion, but scanning the entire slide may be more easily carried out with a $\times 40$ objective. In order not to miss any specimens or fragments from tissue samples, slides must be carefully scanned, moving along transects, covering the entire cover slip. For environmental samples where specimens are likely to be more abundant, it may only be necessary to examine a number of fields of view to determine the species composition of the assemblage. When, on examining a new field of view, the observer no longer finds additional species they probably have a good approximation of the composition, although it is worth scanning along an entire transect to ensure that taxa have not been missed due to any uneven settling on the cover slip. If the microscope has a high resolution digital camera attachment, it is also useful to take images of the different taxa encountered, as a check on, and record of, identifications and to facilitate comparison between different samples.

Diatom assemblages from environmental samples are usually evaluated by counting between 300 and 500 specimens (valves) per sample, recording the number of valves of each and every species encountered. These data are then converted into percentage values for each taxon and comparisons can then be readily made between different samples. The simplest method of assemblage comparison uses similarity tests, which take into account both the species and their relative abundances, for example the Bray-Curtis index (Bray and Curtis, 1957). Using detrended correspondence analysis, Cameron (2004) illustrated how such assemblage data can be presented graphically, in this case revealing that the diatom assemblages taken from the clothing and shoes of a suspect best matched the river mud where a murder victim was found.

The condition of the diatoms in a sample may also be informative. Frustules and valves from actively growing field samples are usually intact and undamaged, whereas damage can be incurred if diatoms have been ingested and then excreted by animals in the ecosystem, subject to mechanical damage after death, or to partial dissolution as for example in sediments (Barker *et al.*, 1990, 1994; Ryves *et al.*, 2001). The longer the period of time since the diatoms were alive, the more likely they are to exhibit some kind of damage or change.

9.7 Reporting and court appearance

Although diatoms can be informative in the diagnosis of death by drowning, this diagnosis can ultimately only be given by a pathologist. Reporting diatom evidence must therefore be carefully worded, bearing in mind that diatoms may be present in a body where drowning is not the cause of death, and that their absence does not necessarily preclude death by drowning (Piette and De Letter, 2006; Pollanen *et al.*, 1997). Where diatoms are being considered as trace evidence (e.g. of presence at a crime scene), demonstrating sample comparability is more straightforward, but it may be necessary to give thought to the way in which the data are presented, bearing in mind that the majority of the population are unfamiliar with diatoms and their biology. In every case, a report should focus on the factual evidence and avoid speculative inference.

Any report must include details of the sample provenance, its preparation for examination and a summary of the findings. The results of an examination would be expected to include the identity, condition and number of diatom specimens in the sample, the type of habitat in which they are normally found, and comments on their condition (i.e. largely intact or damaged). The origin of the diatoms can be inferred, for example the likelihood that they came from water in which a body was found or match specimens on an individual's clothing, and this might include some details on the particular species involved and when they might be expected to be abundant in the field. Similarity of diatom assemblages in the water and/or sediment at the scene and on clothing for instance can quite clearly demonstrate shared provenance, with the use of similarity indices or graphical representation of similarity (Cameron, 2004) helping the non-specialist. In cases of suspected drowning, it may be possible to conclude that diatoms came from the water body in question, but because presence in the body alone does not indicate drowning, diagnosis of death must be left to the forensic pathologist.

Morgan and Bull (2007) discuss some of the potential problems in evaluating trace evidence and the extent to which provenance can be inferred, interestingly suggesting that greater emphasis should be given to excluding, rather than matching, samples. They also provide some precautionary comments on the way in which findings should be presented, arguing that physical evidence and its analysis cannot be wrong, but that error can be introduced in its interpretation.

References

Barber, H.G. and Haworth, E.Y. 1981. *A Guide to the Morphology of the Diatom Frustule*. Freshwater Biological Association, Special Publication No. 44, Ambleside, Cumbria.

Barker, P., Fontes, J.C., Gasse, F. and Druart, J.C. 1994. Experimental dissolution of diatom silica in concentrated salt solutions and implications for palaeoenvironmental reconstruction. *Limnology and Oceanography* **39**: 99–110.

Barker, P., Gasse, F., Roberts, N. and Taieb, M. 1990. Taphonomy and diagenesis in diatom assemblages; a Late Pleistocene palaeoecological study from Lake Magadi, Kenya. *Hydrobiologia* **214**: 267–272.

Battarbee, R.W., Thrush, B.A., Clymo, R.S. *et al.* 1984. Diatom analysis and the acidification of lakes [and discussion]. *Philosophical Transactions of the Royal Society of London B* **305**: 451–477.

Bray, J.R. and Curtis, J.T. 1957. An ordination of the upland forest communities of southern Wisconsin. *Ecological Monographs* **27**: 325–349.

Cameron, N.G. 2004. The use of diatom analysis in forensic geoscience. In K. Pye and D.J. Croft (eds) *Forensic Geoscience: Principles, Techniques and Applications*. Geological Society, Special publications 232, London, pp. 277–280.

Casamatta, D.A. and Verb. R.G. 2000. Algal colonization of submerged carcasses in a mid-order woodland stream. *Journal of Forensic Sciences* **45**: 1280–1285.

Clarke, K.B. 1991. The search for a Norfolk lake deposit containing *Cyclotella*: a cautionary tale and some observations on *C. sevillana* Deby and *C. sexpunctata* Deby. *Diatom Research* **6**: 211–221.

Cox, E.J. 1988. Has the role of the substratum been under-estimated for algal distribution patterns in freshwater ecosystems? *Biofouling* **1**: 49–63.

Cox, E.J. 1990a. Studies on the algae of a small softwater stream. I. Occurrence and distribution with particular reference to the diatoms. *Archiv für Hydrobiologie/Supplement (Monographische Beiträge)* **83**: 525–552.

Cox, E.J. 1990b. Studies on the algae of a small softwater stream. III. Interaction between discharge, sediment composition and diatom flora. *Archiv für Hydrobiologie/Supplement (Monographische Beiträge)* **83**: 567–584.

Cox, E.J. 1990c. Microdistributional patterns of freshwater diatoms in relation to their use as bioindicators. In H. Simola (ed.) *Proceedings of the 10th International Diatom Symposium, Finland 1988*. Koenigstein, Koeltz, pp. 521–528.

Cox, E.J. 1996. *Identification of Freshwater Diatoms from Live Material*. Chapman and Hall, London.

Cox, E.J. 2011. Morphology: cell wall, cytology, ultrastructure and morphogenetic studies. In J. Seckbach and J.P. Kociolek (eds) *The Diatom World*. Series: Cellular Origin, Life in Extreme Habitats and Astrobiology 19. Springer, New York, pp. 21–45.

Harwood, D.M. 2010. Diatomite. In J.P. Smol and F.F. Stoermer (eds) *The Diatoms: Applications for the Environmental and Earth Sciences*, 2nd edn. Cambridge University Press, Cambridge, pp. 570–574.

Horton, B.P. 2007. Diatoms and forensic science. In S. Starratt (ed.) *Pond Scum to Carbon Sink: Geological and Environmental Applications of the Diatoms*. The Paleontological Society Papers 13. The Paleontological Society, USA, pp. 13–22.

Horton. B.P., Boreham, S. and Hillier, C. 2006. The development and application of a diatom-based quantitative reconstruction technique in forensic science. *Journal of Forensic Sciences* **51**: 643–650.

Keiper, J.B. and Casamatta, D.A. 2001. Benthic organisms as forensic indicators. *Journal of the North American Benthological Society* **20**: 311–324.

Kelly, M.G. 2000. *Identification of Common Benthic Diatoms in Rivers*. Field Studies Council, AIDGAP Guides 260, Shrewsbury.

Krammer, K. and Lange-Bertalot, H. 1986. Bacillariophyceae. 1. Teil. Naviculaceae. In H. Ettl, J. Gerloff, H. Heynig and D. Mollenhauer (eds) *Süßwasserflora von Mitteleuropa, Band 2/1*. Gustav Fischer Verlag, Stuttgart.

Krammer, K. and Lange-Bertalot, H. 1988. Bacillariophyceae. 2. Teil. Epithemiaceae, Bacillariophyceae, Surirellaceae. In H. Ettl, J. Gerloff, H. Heynig and D. Mollenhauer (eds) *Süßwasserflora von Mitteleuropa, Band 2/2*. Gustav Fischer Verlag, Stuttgart.

Krammer, K. and Lange-Bertalot, H. 1991a. Bacillariophyceae. 3. Teil. Centrales. In H. Ettl, J. Gerloff, H. Heynig and D. Mollenhauer (eds) *Süßwasserflora von Mitteleuropa, Band 2/3*. Gustav Fischer Verlag, Stuttgart.

Krammer, K. and Lange-Bertalot, H. 1991b. Bacillariophyceae. 4. Teil. Achnanthaceae. In H. Ettl, J. Gerloff, H. Heynig and D. Mollenhauer (eds) *Süßwasserflora von Mitteleuropa, Band 2/4*. Gustav Fischer Verlag, Stuttgart.

Mann, D.G. and Droop, S.J.M. 1996. Biodiversity, biogeography and conservation of diatoms. In J. Kristiansen (ed.) *Biogeography of Freshwater Algae*. *Hydrobiologia* **336**: 19–32.

Moores, S. 2008. Blood, sweat and beers, filtration minerals reviewed. *Industrial Minerals* **484**: 34–40.

Morgan, R.M. and Bull, P.A. 2007. Forensic geoscience and crime detection. Identification, interpretation and presentation in forensic geoscience. *Minerva Medicolegale* **127**: 73–89.

Peabody, A.J. 1999. Forensic science and diatoms. In E.F. Stoermer and J.P. Smol (eds) *The Diatoms: Applications for the Environmental and Earth Sciences*. Cambridge University Press, Cambridge, pp. 413–418.

Peabody, A.J. and Burgess, R.M. 1984. Diatoms in the diagnosis of death by drowning. In D.G. Mann (ed.) *Proceedings of the 7th International Diatom Symposium*. Koenigstein, Koeltz, pp. 537–541.

Peabody, A.J. and Cameron, N.G. 2010. Forensic science and diatoms. In J.P. Smol and E.F. Stoermer (eds) *The Diatoms: Applications for the Environmental and Earth Sciences*, 2nd edn. Cambridge University Press, Cambridge, pp. 534–539.

Piette, M.H.A. and De Letter, E.A. 2006. Drowning: still a difficult autopsy diagnosis. *Forensic Science International* **163**: 1–9.

Pollanen, M.S. 1998. *Forensic Diatomology and Drowning*. Elsevier, Amsterdam.

Pollanen, M.S., Cheung, L. and Chaisson, D.A. 1997. The diagnostic value of the diatom test for drowning. I. Utility: a retrospective analysis of 771 cases of drowning in Ontario, Canada. *Journal of Forensic Sciences* **42**: 281–285.

Reynolds, C.S. 2006. *Ecology of Phytoplankton (Ecology, Biodiversity and Conservation)*. Cambridge University Press, Cambridge.

Round, F.E. 1981. *The Ecology of Algae*. Cambridge University Press, Cambridge.

Round, F.E., Crawford, R.M. and Mann, D.G. 1990. *The Diatoms: Biology and Morphology of the Genera*. Cambridge University Press, Cambridge.

Ryves, D.B., Juggins, S., Fritz, S.C. and Battarbee, R.W. 2001. Experimental diatom dissolution and the quantification of microfossil preservation in sediments. *Palaeogeography, Palaeoclimatology, Palaeoecology* **172**: 93–113.

Siver, P.A., Lord, W.D. and McCarthy, D.J. 1994. Forensic limnology: the use of freshwater algal community ecology to link suspects to an aquatic crime scene in southern New England. *Journal of Forensic Sciences* **39**: 847–853.

Smol, J.P. and Stoermer, E.F. (eds) 2010. *The Diatoms: Applications for the Environmental and Earth Sciences,* 2nd edn. Cambridge University Press, Cambridge.

Sonneman, J., Sincock, A., Fluin, J. *et al.* 2000. *An Illustrated Guide to Common Stream Diatom Species from Temperate Australia.* MDFRC Identification Guide Series 33. CRCFE, Albury, NSW.

Stevenson, R.J., Bothwell, M.L. and Lowe, R.L. 1996. *Algal Ecology. Freshwater Benthic Ecosystems.* Academic Press, San Diego, CA.

Taylor, J.C., Harding, W.R. and Archibald, C.G.M. 2007. *An Illustrated Guide to Some Common Diatom Species from South Africa.* WRC Report TT 282/07. Water Research Commission, Pretoria.

Theriot, E.C., Cannone, J.J., Gutell, R.R. and Alverson, A.J. 2009. The limits of nuclear-encoded SSU rDNA for resolving the diatom phylogeny. *European Journal of Phycology* **44**: 277–290.

Theriot, E.C., Ashworth, M., Ruck. E. *et al.* 2010. A preliminary multigene phylogeny of the diatoms (Bacillariophyta): challenges for future research. *Plant Ecology and Evolution* **143**: 278–296.

Zimmerman, K.A. and Wallace, J.R. 2008. The potential to determine a post-mortem submersion interval based on algal/diatom diversity on decomposing mammalian carcasses in brackish ponds in Delaware. *Journal of Forensic Sciences* **53**: 935–941.

10

Forensic palynology

Beverley Adams-Groom
National Pollen and Aerobiology Research Unit (NPARU), University of Worcester, Worcester, UK

10.1 Introduction and current state of the discipline

Forensic Palynology is the scientific use of pollen, spores and other microscopic biological entities in various crime cases to provide links between suspect and scene or victim and scene. For example, a particular pollen profile on a suspect's footwear might be similar to that found at the deposition site. This chapter deals with the ways in which pollen evidence may be sought and analysed in typical crime cases, particularly in the United Kingdom. The use of palynology as trace evidence is an important subdiscipline of forensic botany which is the subject of Chapter 11.

Palynology is the study of pollen, spores and other microscopic biological entities which together are termed palynomorphs. To be able to assess an enquiry from the police and undertake a full palynological analysis for a case and present the resulting evidence in court, requires the wide range of experience and knowledge of an expert palynologist. However, the information given in this chapter could equip other personnel at a crime scene with sufficient knowledge to understand what to look for and how and where to sample. Most importantly, having personnel with some palynological awareness at a scene *from the beginning* will ensure that important evidence is not lost or destroyed. All too often, palynology is turned to as a last resort and by the time the control samples are collected, the scene can have changed so much that the evidence may be too weak to be of use.

10.1.1 Current state of the discipline

Most forensic companies in the United Kingdom now have forensic palynologists working for them, either in-house or as subcontractors. At the current time of writing, palynology is mainly used in serious crime cases and not for common crimes,

Forensic Ecology Handbook: From Crime Scene to Court, First Edition.
Edited by Nicholas Márquez-Grant and Julie Roberts.
© 2012 John Wiley & Sons, Ltd. Published 2012 by John Wiley & Sons, Ltd.

such as a house burglary. This may be due to costs but could also be due to the fact that palynology, as a fairly recent addition to the forensic arsenal, has low precedence of use in the court system (Bryant and Jones, 2006). In addition, the evidence gained through palynological analysis may often be no more than corroborative and can be superseded by hard evidence such as DNA matching. Molecular methods for matching the DNA of plants themselves are well developed (Craft, Owens and Ashley, 2007; Miller Coyle, 2005) but the development of techniques for matching the DNA of pollen grains or pollen profiles are in their infancy.

Palynology has been used in forensic cases for about 40 years but the main disciplines on which it is based are not new. Pollen morphology and the presence of pollen in the environment have been studied at length by palynologists but forensic palynology also draws on other life science disciplines, particularly ecology and aerobiology (the study of biological particles in the atmosphere). Aerobiology plays an important role in forensic palynology because it aids understanding of the movement, dispersal, seasonality and abundance of pollen and spore types in the environment. In most forensic samples from both the United Kingdom and other parts of the world, the local wind-dispersed types are highly represented while those pollinated by other methods (insects, animals, water, etc.) usually occur infrequently or not at all.

10.2 Pollen

10.2.1 Palynomorphs

Pollen grains come from flowering plants and are essential to the reproduction of most plants and trees. Pollen is just one of a range of microscopic biological entities that can be used as evidence although it is the type most commonly encountered in forensic samples. Other groups include the spores of fungi, moulds, algae, diatoms, ferns and mosses. Palynomorphs can be present in the air, soil and water in varying concentrations. Fungal spores can occasionally be useful as trace evidence but for the most part, the majority of types found are ubiquitous and therefore of little use. Fern spores tend to be site-specific and can be useful in some cases, while many mosses have spores that are very difficult to separate morphologically and it tends to be the presence of moss plants themselves that offer the value.

10.2.2 The uniqueness of pollen

Each pollen grain contains the plant's male gametes (sperm cells) and therefore the male DNA. Certain pollen characteristics have evolved to protect the gametes on their travels, to ensure they reach their destination intact and to allow pollination to occur. As a result each plant genus has its own unique pollen grain morphology that can be identified by the experienced practitioner. In addition, each location will have its own pollen assemblage (also referred to as a pollen profile or pollen fingerprint) based on the type of vegetation present now and in the past. Since pollen grains are microscopic (ranging from approximately 10 to 120 microns in length), are often produced in high numbers by the plants, are tough enough to survive extremes of most kinds, endure in the environment for many years and have good adhesive properties, they can be used as trace evidence in certain criminal cases. The pollen profile of a location can be unique due to a variety of factors such as topography, soil type, land-use, current and past vegetation and climate. In addition, some pollen types are uncommon and their presence can increase the evidential value of an individual pollen profile.

10.2.3 Typical pollen sample profile

Wind-pollinated plants usually have indistinctive, small flowers. Many of them are trees or shrubs and catkins are a typical form for the flowers. The pollen is usually produced in large amounts by these plants, is aerodynamically formed, light, buoyant and with little surface structure. Plant families that have many wind-pollinated types and produce abundant amounts of pollen are well represented in samples, particularly Poaceae (Grasses), Urticaceae (Nettles), Betulaceae (Birches), Pinaceae (Pines and Larches), Fagaceae (Oaks) and Chenopodiaceae (Goosefoots). In the United Kingdom, most samples contain grass pollen and the majority contain birch, nettle, alder and pine. Some types of wind-pollinated plants produce lower amounts of pollen or have heavier pollen grains which do not travel far and are therefore more site-specific. Examples of these include Juglandaceae (Walnuts), Platanaceae (Planes), Aceraceae (Maples), Plantaginaceae (Plantains) and Polygonaceae (Knotweeds and Docks).

Insect-pollinated plants tend to have attractive flowers, their pollen is usually produced in smaller amounts than wind-pollinated types, has more surface structure and often a sticky substance is present on the grains, called pollenkitt, which enables it to be collected deliberately or in passing by insects, birds and other animals. The pollen from insect-pollinated plants is usually removed from the location by the insects/animals or falls directly to the ground beneath, or surrounding, the plant. For this reason, insect-pollinated plants and their pollen tend to be location-specific and, in addition, those types that also have restricted habitats can therefore be particularly useful in identifying a site or linking an item or suspect to a crime scene. The disadvantage, however, is that the low concentrations of these pollen types in soil samples means that very few of the grains will be transferred to an exhibit or be present on a body or other item and this can make the evidence weak unless the rest of the profile bears a strong resemblance overall to the control samples.

Some plants have pollen that is dispersed by both insects and wind. They tend to have attractive flowers but with anthers exposed to the airstream. These types are often frequently found in samples and include the following families: Rosaceae (Roses, Cherries, Apples), Salicaceae (Willows), Ericaceae (Heathers), Brassicaceae (Cabbage family – especially Oil-seed rape in the United Kingdom) and some members of the Asteraceae (Daisy family) such as *Centaurea* (Knapweed), *Achillea* (Yarrow) and *Artemisia* (Mugwort).

The presence of pollen from aquatic plants, or the whole or parts of the plants themselves, can be very useful in a forensic sample as they are habitat-specific. However, although the majority of types are either insect-pollinated or their pollen is dispersed by water, some are wind-dispersed and can be found at a distance from the source. *Typha* (Reedmace) is a typical example and its presence in a sample of a few percent would indicate that the sample could have come from a site either in the vicinity of an aquatic habitat or actually from it. It could also indicate that the soil containing this pollen type has been flooded by a watercourse containing *Typha*. Pollen from other types of aquatic plants would be necessary in the profile to suggest it had actually come from such a habitat.

10.2.4 Pollen morphology

Pollen grains have four main characteristics used for identification: size, shape, apertures and ornamentation and much more detail on these aspects can be obtained in, for example, Moore, Webb and Collinson (1991) or Faegri and Iversen (1989). Figure 10.1 shows examples of palynomorphs (pollen, spores and fern spores).

10.2.5 Moulds, fungi and algae

Fungal spores are produced by fungi either vegetatively or sexually and can be difficult to identify to species level in many cases. Their forms are variable but they all have a structured wall and the vast majority are in the size range 2–200 microns. Although many types of spores from moulds and fungi are often found very commonly in samples, some types are very specific to a location. Rotting wood and decaying faeces, in particular, can harbour such types and even if the moulds themselves may not be visible it is worth sampling these substrates if a suspect could have walked on them. An expert mycologist is usually required to identify fungal spores. In some samples, an abundance of a particular spore type may be of interest, particularly those from mushrooms or toadstools that only grow in certain habitats.

Algae occur in damp places, such as shallow standing water, as well as in rivers, ponds and lakes and may provide useful trace evidence but careful processing must be done to obtain the algae.

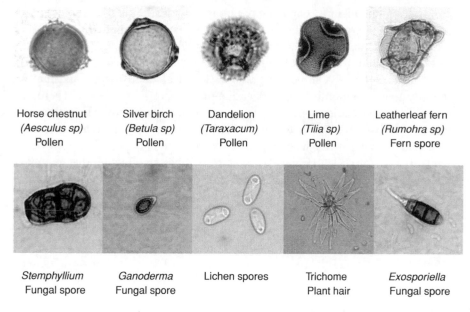

| Horse chestnut (Aesculus sp) Pollen | Silver birch (Betula sp) Pollen | Dandelion (Taraxacum) Pollen | Lime (Tilia sp) Pollen | Leatherleaf fern (Rumohra sp) Fern spore |

| Stemphyllium Fungal spore | Ganoderma Fungal spore | Lichen spores | Trichome Plant hair | Exosporiella Fungal spore |

Figure 10.1 A selection of palynomorphs.

10.2.6 Mosses and ferns

Although it is difficult to identify many moss spores to species or genus level, for the most part, the spores of Sphagnum moss can be identified and can be site-specific as they largely occur in damp habitats such as marshy ground, peatbogs and woodlands. However, they are also present in peat used for planting in gardens and parks so their presence in a sample should be treated with caution.

Ferns grow mainly in damp, shady areas but some types, such as polyplody grow on walls in urban areas and bracken can grow in quite dry soil (on fairly acidic soils). Since ferns are largely site-specific, their presence in a sample can be important and many types have distinctive spores that are readily identified. However, the chemical processing used to separate the soil matrix from the palynomorphs must be done carefully to avoid removing the outer coat (perine) of some types of fern spore as this is an important feature in identification.

10.2.7 Distribution of pollen and spores within soil

Pollen rains down onto the soil in various ways. It may fall directly from the plant above, drift from nearby plants, or arrive on air currents from further away. Birch trees, for example, produce millions of pollen grains per tree so the pollen tends to be over-represented in samples and can be present in a sample even though there are no birch trees in the vicinity. Once the pollen is in the soil, it is then subject to the actions of soil fauna, particularly worms, which consume the pollen grains which then pass through their bodies (Davidson *et al.*, 1999). This can happen repeatedly to a pollen grain and over time it can be deposited deeper into the soil and become damaged in the process. The pollen grain wall will gradually erode and may be attacked by fungi leading to further degradation (Moore *et al.*, 1991). Therefore, the grains in best condition will tend to be on the surface from recent pollen rain and older types will be deeper down. Pollen grains will also increase in size as they age and the integrity of their structure weakens. It is not possible, however, to determine the age of pollen grains. The type of soil has an effect on the amount of pollen to be found in a sample. Rich brown soils full of humus will usually contain high concentrations of pollen but the more gritty and sandy the soil, the lower the concentrations due to leaching. It is usually worth examining the mineral content of the soil as well as the palynomorphs as this can often strengthen the evidential value of the match between exhibit samples and control samples.

10.2.8 Pollen assemblages

Each type of outdoor habitat will have its own unique palynological assemblage which will be composed of some or all of the following: palynomorphs from local plants and fungi; pollen from plants that have recently flowered; pollen that has blown in from external sources; palynomorphs from plants/fungi that previously grew at the location but are no longer present. A habitat can be very small and may be isolated (e.g. flower bed, small pond, copse) or larger (e.g. oak woodland, crop field, hedgerow, heathland). Within the latter, there is very likely to be micro-habitats that should be sampled too. For example, in a beech woodland, with an overall ground cover of bluebells and dog's mercury, there may be some wetter areas where plants that prefer damp conditions grow, such as knotweed or balsam, for example. Every individual habitat where a suspect could have picked up pollen or where a vehicle could have been driven, should have a control sample taken from it because the pollen there could have contributed to the general pollen profile present on an exhibit.

10.3 Applications

There are four main categories of application for palynological analysis:

- **Relating a suspect or item to a crime scene or victim:** Plants, or parts of plants such as leaves, stems, flowers, seeds, and pollen can be used to provide a link between suspect or victim and crime scene. Soil samples can be taken from the clothing and footwear of victims, suspects, vehicles or other pertinent items and these can be analysed for palynomorphs and compared to scene control samples.

- **Estimating season of death or last time of exposure (e.g. documents, weapons, body):** The growth rates of plants can suggest a time period or season (e.g. where growth of plants has occurred over a clandestine grave), while decay rates of vegetation can offer similar information. The profile of pollen on a body (e.g. in the hair, under the fingernails, in the nasal cavities) or on an item can indicate season of death or last exposure if the body has not been opened to the ambient air in the intervening period of time.

- **Narrowing a search area to locate a grave, body or scene:** Plant parts and palynomorphs can be used to indicate a locality or location, particularly if a profile of plants is found. Typically, a profile would be obtained from a vehicle or footwear. The presence of plant parts on a body that are alien to the location where a body is found could suggest the body has been moved from another location.

- **Tracing an item to a source (e.g. drugs, documents, weapons, money or counterfeit goods):** The pollen profile on an item can indicate whereabouts it has come from. It is often surprising how many palynomorphs can be found on items that look clean. For example, in one case the authorities wanted to know where counterfeit condoms may be originating. There were various layers of packaging for analysis, such as the outer cardboard transportation boxes, the retailers' packets and the cellophane wrapper of the consumer packet itself, all of which looked 'clean'. Pollen was found in most of the samples taken and China was identified as the country of origin.

10.3.1 Case example: narrowing a search area and linking items to a scene

A man was murdered and the suspect was his lover's husband but no body had been found. The police had sampled soil from inside and outside of the victim's vehicle thought to have been used to deposit the body. Pollen analysis showed a woodland profile composed particularly of sycamore, lime tree, sweet chestnut, dog's mercury and bracken fern. Following intelligence information and the pollen profile, a number of woodlands were examined in the area and one, which matched this profile, was found to contain a wheelbarrow (later confirmed to belong to the suspect) and two spades, the latter of which were sampled for pollen. Eventually, the body was located in an unusually deep grave (underlying a sweet chestnut tree) from which control samples were taken. The soil from the spades contained unusually high concentrations of sweet chestnut pollen and bracken spores and best matched the pollen profile of the sample taken from the deepest part of the grave, indicating that they had been used to dig it. The soil found within the driver's foot-well of the vehicle also had a good match with the grave area. In addition, of a choice of three possible parking locations in which the vehicle could have been parked at the woodland, the overall car pollen profile best matched the one located nearest to where the grave was eventually found.

10.4   Pre-scene attendance

A visit to a crime scene or an associated site by a forensic palynologist usually involves initial discussions with the crime scene manager (CSM) handling the case. Police budgets tend to be tight and palynology is often only turned to when other forensic avenues have proved negative. It is highly recommended that the scene is documented as soon as possible by the expert who may notice aspects of it that are either useful in evidential terms or which can eliminate the use of palynology in the case. To avoid wasting police time and money on analysis that may not be of any use, it is important to establish the points below:

- What precisely do the police want to determine and can palynology actually help to achieve this? In most cases, palynology can only offer supporting evidence.

- Tying suspect to a location: in a case where the police want to establish whether or not someone was present at a particular scene, it is important to understand the habitat of that location and whether or not the person could have spent time in similar habitats (e.g. Does the person work outdoors, walk a dog in the vicinity of the location or visit similar locations?).

- Season of death: Would it be reasonable to assume that the body has remained covered from the ambient air since death occurred? If not, then there is probably no point in pursuing palynological analysis.

- In the United Kingdom, many areas have largely homogenous flora which would not yield a pollen profile unique enough to be of use. There either needs to be some site-specific plants that have transferrable pollen, plantings of exotic trees and shrubs, a habitat that is uncommon in the area of the crime (e.g. a patch of heathland in an arable landscape) and/or a diverse pollen/spore assemblage due to a combination of habitats in one location.

- Length of time since crime occurred and sampling for pollen: over time the pollen profile of a location will change so the chances of obtaining good pollen comparator samples decreases the longer it is since the crime occurred. However, where a body has been found in a grave, it may still be possible to gather useful evidence from in and around the body, even after many years, depending on where the body has been located.

In some instances the possibility of getting useful evidence may be slim so it is important to try to give an estimate of the likely strength of the outcome to the police to allow them to decide whether or not they wish to continue.

10.5   Scene attendance

Since palynology is not always the first priority at a crime scene, this type of evidence can often be damaged or lost by the need to gather other forms of forensic evidence. Ideally, a palynologist will be called out to the scene immediately. However, this is not always possible logistically or in terms of cost. Therefore, the scene needs to be photographed as soon as possible before any clearance or removal of scene items. In many cases, this will be done by the police photographer but regardless of who undertakes this task, very detailed photographs of any vegetation at the scene should be taken. Obviously, in winter time there will be less vegetation but there may be mosses or branches growing over a grave, for example. Perhaps there are branches that have been cut and these can be photographed in detail too. Although Scenes of Crime Officers can collect scene control samples if they have some botanical knowledge, or have consulted a relevant specialist, there is no substitute for getting an experienced person onto the site where important information may become apparent that is not obvious to others.

10.5.1   Summary of the process of a scene visit

Below are some useful bullet points regarding the protocol or process when attending a scene:

- Scene assessment with the Police Officers who will discuss the approach and provide information about the scene and the case.

- Survey of vegetation contained in and around the site to indicate the likely pollen assemblage.

- Samples may be collected for pollen or botanical analysis.

- Scene evaluation to determine whether or not palynological analysis is worth pursuing and whether or not other locations should also be visited.

- Possible requirement to attempt to seek the location of a clandestine grave.

- Possible visits to other locations from which control samples are to be obtained (similar treatment to main scene required).

- Possible mortuary and/or car pound visit to collects samples.

10.5.2   Details of scene attendance: surveying and sample collection

10.5.2.1   Assessment of site(s)

Each scene/site and case is different and the approach will depend on what the police want to determine, how many sites need to be visited and the amount of time available to do so, the topography of and access to the scene/site, the season and the weather. The assessment of the site may result in the expert deciding that pollen analysis will not be useful in this case or, conversely, it may lead to the need to access and assess other locations.

On arrival at the scene, the expert will discuss with the police what is required to be done and will then decide how to proceed. If a body is present or the area has only recently been cordoned off, then the scene will be tightly controlled by the police and the palynologist must pay careful attention to the integrity of the scene, wear protective clothing if appropriate and follow police instructions. Vegetation is often removed from a scene by the police to enable a fingertip search so it may be necessary to request a delay until notes have been made and samples collected.

10.5.2.2 Plan of site

Using grid paper, a plan of the site can be made, including a grid reference, and a compass should be used to identify North. Particular features and the locations of the pollen samples should be noted on the plan. Ideally, the scene should be divided into sections pertinent to the different areas of vegetation and each section given a name or code (Figure 10.2). This will help to identify areas later during the report stage. In some cases, the scene may already have been divided into a grid or sections by the police, in which case that layout should be followed.

10.5.2.3 Vegetation survey

For each different habitat area or location and the surrounding area of the scene, the vegetation should be noted and a comment included on the abundance of each

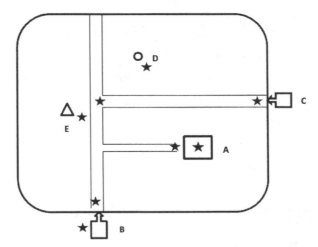

Figure 10.2 Example of a basic scene survey plan for an enclosed woodland. A: deposition site; B: possible parking area and entry location; C: alternative possible entry location; D: location of found weapon; E: location of found mobile phone; ★ location of control samples.

type. At a later date, the survey can be written up tidily into a report with the plants in standard order, that is, Trees and Shrubs, Herbaceous types, etc. If working for the defence, the palynologist may be attending a scene that the defendant claims to have visited. In which case, there will be a list of pollen/plant types prepared from the crime scene to compare to the current location. It is very important to check the wider area of a scene for types that may not be present at the immediate location. Any plants that cannot be identified on site should be wrapped in tissue or paper to aid preservation and put into clearly labelled brown paper bags. Vegetation samples should later be stored in a warm, dry place. High resolution photographs should be taken of all vegetation, particularly around the deposition site and at entry and exit points if relevant.

Where plants are growing over a body or clandestine grave, these should be measured, photographed and detailed notes taken of their appearance. Plant parts used to cover a grave (e.g. twigs, logs, leaves) can be taken as exhibits for later analysis. These can be examined to determine species, length of time since they were cut or broken from the plant and decay rates due to fungal activity.

10.5.2.4 Indoor scene

Occasionally there may be the need to sample indoors, where a suspect could have brushed past houseplants for example, in which case a sample of the flower's anthers should be taken for the pollen. Detailed photographs should be taken of houseplants. Carpets or other surfaces can be sampled for soil deposits and other dust or debris that could contain palynomorphs.

10.5.2.5 Contamination of samples

At all stages of collection and analysis for forensic palynology, there should be an awareness of the potential for the ambient air to contaminate the sample, particularly during the spring and summer. There is also the risk of cross-contamination between samples.

10.5.2.6 Collection of samples

There may be a number of different locations or habitats from which to take control samples, including access points or paths if relevant. In most cases, the samples will be controls but it may also be necessary to take exhibit samples at the scene, for example if there is a body present. Most soil samples should be collected from the top few millimetres of soil and *no deeper* and from a representative area of the soil type (up to 1–2 metres wide). Gloves should be worn when collecting samples and about $4\,cm^3$ should be taken and placed in a sterile tube or pot, taking a greater amount of sample from sandy soil as pollen is poorly represented in this type. A plant label can be used to mark the location and then it can be noted on the site plan. Full forensic overalls, face mask, goggles and double gloves should be worn when collecting from a grave and any samples collected from in or around a body should be placed in tight containers and placed in a small plastic bag, labelled, and then put into a Biohazard evidence bag. Samples from a grave should be taken from the different layers of soil within it, a sample of the spoil which will have a mixture of the different soil layers, a sample from underneath the body or directly beside it and one from where it is likely the suspect stood within the grave when digging out the deepest layer.

There may be other types of surface from which to gather samples: leaf litter; lawn; plants which could have rubbed/pressed against clothing; surface with algae on; dust from a ledge, windowsill, seat, etc. It may be necessary to wash a surface to obtain a sample using a solution of distilled water and 3 % detergent and scrub with a toothbrush (different one for each sample) or use nylon swabs if a gentle action is required, or the area is small. Check with the Crime Scene Manager (CSM) that such samples can be taken as other evidence may be needed from the same surface (e.g. fingerprints or DNA samples).

10.5.3   Sampling a suspect, living victim or body

Footwear usually yields the best pollen evidence as it can collect soil directly from where the suspect has trodden. The deeper the tread, the more soil it is likely to have collected. Soil, pollen and other botanical items can also be collected from clothing, for example from lower parts of trousers and areas that have rubbed on soil. Folding clothing up can redistribute palynomorphs across a garment so the item should be dealt with in a suitable way. Samples can also be collected from hair and under nails. The best way to obtain pollen samples is by scraping off the soil and/or by washing with a warm detergent solution and a toothbrush, then centrifuging the liquid to obtain a pellet. Plant parts are sometimes caught in footwear, clothing, in hair or under nails and the person should be checked for these too. Similar samples can be collected from a body to those of suspects and living victims but the nasal cavities can also be sampled for the pollen gathered in the last breath if the nose is likely to have remained covered since death. Details of this process can be found in Wiltshire and Black (2006). In cases where sexual assault is implicated, then sampling the vaginal area and buttocks for palynomorphs may also be necessary.

10.5.4   Sampling a vehicle

Since the majority of cars are never taken off-road, soil on the outside of a vehicle can be significant (Brown, Smith and Elmhurst, 2002). Soil samples can be collected from wheels, wheel arches, foot pedals, foot-wells and the car boot if relevant. Each area should be treated as a separate sample and if there are visibly different soil types, these should be sampled individually.

10.5.5   Storage of soil samples

Soil samples should be stored in a fridge and any samples that are very wet or contain body fluids should be frozen until required.

10.6   Mortuary attendance

Mortuary attendance is rarely required for palynological analysis of a body but will usually require sampling similar to that of a scene, such as sampling the nasal cavities and looking for pieces of vegetation. The pathologist will discuss the requirements for botanical analysis and lead the work. All kit required by the botanist/palynologist should be taken along as the required sampling items are unlikely to be available. The air should be monitored for contamination by palynomorphs, ideally with a volumetric air sampler.

10.7   Laboratory analysis

Once the samples or exhibits have been received, they will normally first be examined and notes taken and then, in the case of soil samples, processed for palynomorphs, or, in the case of an item, washed, swabbed or taped. Washing or swabbing is the best way to obtain a pollen sample but in certain cases taping or vacuuming with a filter may be the only way to proceed without compromising the item or other evidence. The samples are then ready for chemical separation of the palynomorphs from the soil matrix. The standard extraction processes for pollen and spores for forensic purposes are acetolysis and heavy liquid separation which are detailed in Brown (2008). Different methods are used for diatoms (see Chapter 9). After processing there should be a small pellet in the base of the test tube which can then be either carefully mixed with mountant and put onto a slide for light microscopy or onto a stub for electron microscopy.

10.7.1   Identification and counting of palynomorphs

It is usually necessary to quantify the pollen and other palynomorphs present in a sample. There are no automated systems sophisticated enough at the time of writing to determine the often subtle differences within and between pollen types, so microscopy (light, scanning electron or transmission electron) remains the best way to achieve identification. Ideally, a minimum of 300 grains are counted in each sample to allow percentage concentrations to be compared between them. However, if a particular type dominates the profile it may be necessary to count more to ensure that the rarer types are picked up. The amount needed very much depends on the type of sample and the type of evidence that is being sought. It is not always necessary to count all of every sample if it becomes clear during the process that the profile is very similar or rather dissimilar to that of the control samples. Once the data has been collected they are entered onto a spreadsheet. If the results require comparisons between two sets of samples, for example the suspect's footwear compared to grave samples, the data can be converted to percentages to compare the relative frequencies of the types. The percentages can then be compared using statistics that compare similarity of abundance for the types in common, using, for example, the Czekanowski coefficient. In some cases, cluster analysis may also be useful.

10.7.2   Analysis and interpretation of pollen and spore data

It is very important during the analysis and interpretation of the data not to over-emphasize the presence of the less common types when comparing samples from exhibits with control samples. Honeysuckle (*Lonicera spp*), for example, has large, sticky pollen that is only found where the plant grows. However, honeysuckle is common and occurs in lots of samples so its presence in trace amount in a pollen profile from an item may not be significant because it could, quite easily, have been picked up elsewhere. Other key types would need to be present in both assemblages, in similar proportions, if the results are to be considered of interest to the case.

10.8   Reporting and court appearance

Since palynological evidence is often complex to present, it is important that a very clear interpretation of it is given in the report that the lay person can understand. Where possible, the evidence should be presented clearly in tables or charts, particularly those that show comparisons. Should the evidence be required in court, it is likely that the report will be sent to a palynologist/botanical expert working for the opposing counsel for review which it may be necessary to respond to. There may also be the requirement to visit an alibi scene. In one case example where two suspects had been accused of an aggravated burglary at a farm with a particularly rich and diverse pollen and spore profile, one defendant had stated that he regularly visited another farm some miles away. The other farm was therefore attended but it was clear from the vegetation survey that about 50 % of the pollen types (including most of the site-specific ones) found at the crime scene were not present at the other farm and a number of key types were not present in the surrounding area either.

Before submitting a report that could potentially be used as evidence, the following should be checked:

- Exactly how were the samples collected? Incorrectly collected samples can invalidate the whole evidence.

- Was the scene visited by the expert witness or were very detailed and informative photographs and notes of it received? Visiting a scene and its locality is usually invaluable for informing palynological casework.

- Is it possible that the suspect had a legitimate reason for visiting the scene at some point in the recent past?

- Did the suspect spend time in a similar habitat? People who work outdoors can collect a variety of soil types on their footwear and on or in their cars and clothing. Such profiles could bear a similarity to the crime scene.

- Have similar scenes been sampled or at least visited by the palynologist?

- Could the samples have become contaminated in any way during collection or processing? It is important to know how samples were collected.

These are the sort of points that the opposing counsel will pick up on in court so it is very important that they have been covered during the analysis.

References

Brown, A.G., Smith, A. and Elmhurst, O. 2002. The combined use of pollen and soil analyses in a search and subsequent murder investigation. *Journal of Forensic Sciences* **47**: 614–618.

Brown, C. 2008. *Palynological Techniques*, 2nd edn (J.B. Riding and S. Warny (eds)). American Association of Stratigraphic Palynologists Foundation, Dallas, TX.

Bryant, V.M. and Jones, G.D. 2006. Forensic palynology: Current status of a rarely used technique in the United States of America. *Forensic Science International* **163**: 183–197.

Craft, K.J., Owens, J.D. and Ashley, M.V. 2007. Application of plant DNA marker in forensic botany: Genetic comparison of Quercus evidence leaves to crime scene trees using microsatellites. *Forensic Science International* **165**: 64–70.

Davidson, D.A., Carter, S., Boag, B. *et al.* 1999. Analysis of pollen in soils: processes of incorporation and redistribution of pollen in five soil profile types. *Soil Biology & Biochemistry* **31**: 643–653.

Faegri, K. and Iversen, J. 1989. *Textbook of Pollen Analysis*. John Wiley & Sons, Ltd, Chichester.

Miller Coyle, H. (ed.) 2005. *Forensic Botany: Principles and Applications to Criminal Casework*. CRC Press, Boca Raton, FL.

Moore, P.D., Webb, J.A. and Collinson, M.E. 1991. *Pollen Analysis*, 2nd edn. Blackwell Scientific Publications, Oxford.

Wiltshire, P.E.J. and Black, S. 2006. The cribriform approach to the retrieval of palynological evidence from the turbinates of murder victims. *Forensic Science International* **163**: 224–230.

11

Forensic botany

Heather Miller Coyle, Peter Massey and Peter Valentin
Forensic Science Department, Henry C. Lee College of Criminal Justice and Forensic Sciences, University of New Haven, West Haven, CT, USA

11.1 Introduction

Crime scenes are extremely interesting but very variable in nature. Outdoor and indoor crime scenes, and both primary and secondary scenes, can hold a myriad of trace plant materials including grasses, leaves, pollen, drug samples and food items. The body itself is a crime scene where pollen can be trapped in clothing or on shoes; food can be located in the mouth and digestive tract and leaves are often found attached to hair or blankets surrounding the body. Forensic botany is the application of botany, the classification and individualisation of plants, to matters of law (Miller Coyle, 2005). The aspects of this field of study that can be useful in criminal investigation involve specialised knowledge in plant anatomy, plant growth and behaviour, plant reproductive cycles and population structure, DNA and bioinformatics classification schemes (Miller Coyle, 2005). The goal of this chapter is to provide a broad overview of forensic botany with a focus on crime scene, mortuary, laboratory tests and court acceptance, with particular examples from the United States.

11.2 Applications

Casework examples where plant evidence has been recovered and examinations have been requested include the following: determination of pre-meditation of homicide by leaf accumulation in pre-dug graves; determination of the total number of *Cannabis* samples recovered from a grow site to associate a stiffer court penalty; identification of plant seeds from a blanket used to conceal a body; association of

Forensic Ecology Handbook: From Crime Scene to Court, First Edition.
Edited by Nicholas Márquez-Grant and Julie Roberts.
© 2012 John Wiley & Sons, Ltd. Published 2012 by John Wiley & Sons, Ltd.

grass stains on clothing with a potential sexual assault scene; evaluation of stomach contents for a victim's last meal as an investigative lead to find witnesses at a restaurant; linkage of a tree sample from the barrel of a gun to a tree platform where a stalker was hiding; attempt to link leaf samples from a body found in a dumpster to a defendant's vehicle; and profiling of leaf litter to locate the body of a victim in a murder-suicide (Miller Coyle, 2005). These are just a few examples of how forensic botany can play a useful role in crime scene investigation.

11.3 Pre-scene attendance

Pre-scene preparation begins well before notification of a crime scene is received by an investigator (Gaensslen, Harris and Lee, 2008; Saferstein, 2009; Girard, 2011). The greatest forensic laboratory personnel cannot identify that magical item of evidence if it is not sent to the laboratory for analysis. It is entirely incumbent upon the crime scene investigator to locate all pertinent items of evidence. The working knowledge of what types of evidence may be found at a crime scene is therefore vitally important (Miller Coyle, 2005; Girard, 2011; Allgeier *et al.*, 2011). This would also include transient and conditional evidence (Gaensslen *et al.*, 2008; Saferstein, 2009; Girard, 2011). Transient evidence is evidence that is temporary or is easily lost. Generally, this would be something like smells or odours. In the realm of botanical evidence, it could relate to pollen (see Chapter 10). Conditional evidence is situational. An example of this would be grass stains on clothing or on a body that had been dragged (Gaensslen *et al.*, 2008; Saferstein, 2009; Girard, 2011). The investigator with the mindset that botanical evidence might be located needs to be prepared with proper tools to accurately document the crime scene, specifically where the various items of evidence are located. Proper collection containers, to include, but not be limited to, appropriate-sized paper bags, coin envelopes, druggist folds and containers to hold liquids and solid trace materials are critical (Gaensslen *et al.*, 2008; Saferstein, 2009; Girard, 2011). DNA collection cards can also be used to collect samples for later DNA bar-coding to species and sample level (Allgeier *et al.*, 2011). Tamper evident sealing material (evidence tape) is required to ensure integrity (Gaensslen *et al.*, 2008; Saferstein, 2009; Girard, 2011).

The knowledge of 'Locard's Principle of Exchange' is an inherent educational tool that should be applied in all cases involving the potential for botanical evidence (Gaensslen *et al.*, 2008; Saferstein, 2009; Girard, 2011). Much of this type of evidence is trace in nature (Hunter, 2006; Schierenbeck, 2003; Miller Coyle *et al.*, 2001, 2005; Brown, 2006; Laposata, 1985). Trace evidence includes many types of materials which are transferred as a result of direct contact or deposited in small quantities on an object, victim and suspect or at the scene. The length of time for contact and the circumstances of deposit are factors in how much evidence is transferred from one object to another. It is also possible to have secondary transfer from item to item inherent at the scene or as contamination if proper evidence guidelines are not followed (Gaensslen *et al.*, 2008; Saferstein, 2009; Girard, 2011).

11.4 Scene attendance

The ability to recognise, document and collect evidence is the full function of the crime scene investigator. Once the evidence has been recognised it is vital to indicate, both for chain of custody reasons and for reconstruction purposes, should it be necessary, to document exactly where these evidentiary items were located (Gaensslen *et al.*, 2008; Saferstein, 2009; Girard, 2011). Notes should be made of all activities and locations of all evidence. The entire scene should be video-recorded to allow for those not present to view the scene in its entirety. This will permit a three-dimensional perspective of the scene and the evidence locations to be documented. Individual photographs of the entire scene as well as the specific items of evidence should be taken. Included in the photo series should be close-up, mid-range and distance photos indicating an overall perspective of the individual items. Each item of evidence should be photographed utilising a number marker and a scale where the size of the item is paramount. The final step of documentation would be to measure and sketch every item of evidence that is collected as well as the entire dimension of the scene itself (Figure 11.1). This is to allow for a reconstruction of the crime scene should it be necessary (Gaensslen *et al.*, 2008; Saferstein, 2009; Girard, 2011).

Collection methods vary with each particular item (Gaensslen *et al.*, 2008; Saferstein, 2009; Girard, 2011). Starting with a deceased victim, permission should be obtained from the medical examiner or coroner prior to any collection of evidentiary samples. Once that has been obtained and properly documented, a visual

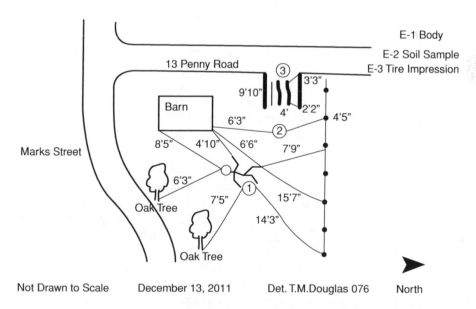

Figure 11.1 Crime scene sketch. Example showing location of vegetation.

inspection of potential botanical evidence should be made. These need to be collected with sterile forceps and properly placed in a druggist's fold acting as a primary container prior to placement in a coin envelope. For those items that are not
easily observed, the use of a lint roller to carefully roll over the victim and/or their
clothing is advisable prior to placement into a body bag. These roller sheets are then
packaged in a paper bag and submitted to the forensic lab for further analysis. Large
tape lifts, gel lifters, or contact paper can be substituted for the lint roller (Gaensslen
et al., 2008; Saferstein, 2009; Girard, 2011; Barash, Reshef and Brauner, 2010). The
use of the aforementioned collection mediums can also be utilised for other items
located at the scene and the scene itself.

The use of vacuuming can be utilised when no visible trace evidence is present
but only use this method after all other collection processes have been used (Miller
Coyle, 2005). This is not a favourite of the forensic examiner and truly should be
used as a last resort due to the possibility of damage to the evidence during the
vacuuming process. Brushing can be used after the obvious trace evidence has been
removed. Brushings should be done over a clean sheet of paper to catch whatever
trace particles are dislodged. In the event that botanical transfer evidence, such as
grass stains, has adhered to clothing the use of cuttings of the stained area may be
preferred.

Soil or botanical evidence may be typically found in shoes, clothing and other
articles associated with a suspect or victim (Miller Coyle, 2005; Hunter, 2006;
Schierenbeck, 2003; Miller Coyle *et al.*, 2001, 2005; Brown, 2006). The outer layer
of clothing items, the pockets, cuffs, folds and collars are areas where minute quantities of trace evidence can be found (Laposata, 1985; Barash *et al.*, 2010). The entire footwear item including the sole, as well as tyres from a motor vehicle should
also be searched. Additionally, many motor vehicles are equipped with air filters for
both the combustible engine and the interior cabin. These should be collected and
sent to the lab for further analysis for pollen, plant particulates and possible DNA
(Miller Coyle, 2005; Allgeier *et al.*, 2011; Walsh and Horrocks, 2008; Mildenhall,
Wiltshire and Bryant, 2006; Mildenhall, 2006a,b; Wu *et al.*, 2006; Ferri *et al.*, 2009,
2012; Bruni *et al.*, 2010; Ward *et al.*, 2005, 2009; Howard *et al.*, 2009; Stambuk
et al., 2007; Virtanen, Korpelainen and Kostamo, 2007; Craft, Owens and Ashley,
2007; Kress *et al.*, 2005). Locations in the wheel wells or under the fenders should
also be examined, as well as other parts of the undercarriage. Plant material is commonly caught in or on vehicles and can be potentially used to link a vehicle to
a scene of a motor vehicle accident or a vehicle to a secondary scene where the
body has been dumped (Figures 11.2a,b). Whenever possible, the article with soil
or botanical evidence should be submitted *in situ* to the lab or the area with the
soil should be cut out if the object is too large to transport (Gaensslen *et al.*, 2008;
Saferstein, 2009; Girard, 2011).

If removing soil evidence, care should be taken to retain the soil layers intact
while packaging and transporting. If the soil is on the suspect's or victim's clothing,
the clothing should be packed in paper, with additional paper between any folds or
layers. If any items that are to be collected are wet with blood, other body fluids,
precipitation or contain any type of moisture, it is imperative to allow them to air

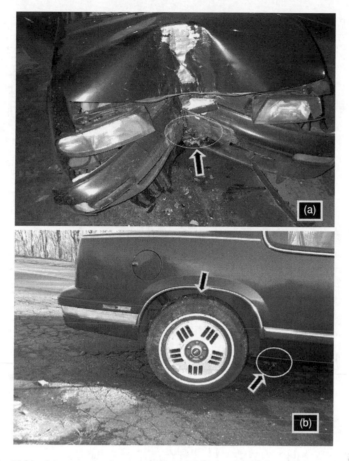

Figure 11.2 Vehicular scenes and vegetation. (a) Linkage of vehicle to a scene with a portion of a tree embedded in front area of vehicle. (b) Grass samples attached to wheels, wheel wells and undercarriage of the vehicle. Both photographs illustrate how a vehicle can be associated back to a scene by vegetative matter.

dry at room temperature. Drying must not be accelerated using a fan or heater. Any items of clothing should be clearly labelled and identified and packaged in paper or in a paper evidence bag using additional paper between the folds as needed. Often, botanical evidence might be in the form of branches, sticks, twigs or similar. If these are determined to be of evidentiary value, they should be packed in an appropriately sized paper bag or rolled in Kraft paper (Miller Coyle, 2005; Gaensslen *et al.*, 2008; Saferstein, 2009; Girard, 2011).

Known control samples are extremely important for proper lab analysis (Miller Coyle 2005). Several samples should be collected from the suspect area or crime scene. These are needed for later comparison to the evidence. Collection cards can be used to take rubbings of plant material from evidence if of sufficient quantity and from known reference plants from the scene for later DNA analysis by STR or sequencing technology (Miller Coyle, 2005; Allgeier *et al.*, 2011). This is a relatively

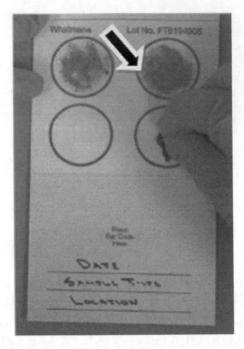

Figure 11.3   Collection cards for DNA analysis of plant material.

new sampling methodology but highly beneficial as the DNA will not degrade over time if placed on these cards. In addition, these cards have anti-fungal and anti-bacterial properties that will prevent growth of organisms which could potentially affect the quality of DNA (Figure 11.3).

11.5   Mortuary attendance

Whenever possible, the forensic scientist should examine the decedent at the scene for potential plant material because evidence that is not recognised and collected cannot be used to advance the investigation (Miller Coyle, 2005; Gaensslen *et al.*, 2008; Saferstein, 2009; Girard, 2011). Since the body is generally the jurisdiction of the medical examiner or forensic pathologist, any examination of the body at the scene should be done only after consultation and collaboration with personnel from the medical examiner.

Quite often, the circumstances surrounding the death under investigation can only be fully understood when information from the scene is combined with the information gleaned from the post-mortem examination. There should be personnel from the investigating agency present at every autopsy. If attendance is not possible at every examination, it should be mandatory in those cases where the potential for plant evidence, or any other trace evidence, is anticipated. When considering the transient nature of trace evidence in general and the potential for plant evidence specifically to be lost or otherwise unrecognised, it becomes paramount to gather potential evidence at the earliest time possible (Laposata, 1985; Barash *et al.*, 2010).

The search for potential plant evidence should begin with the shrouding or bag that was used to transport the body to the medical examiner or forensic pathologist (Miller Coyle, 2005; Miller Coyle *et al.*, 2005; Schierenbeck, 2003; Brown, 2006). Plant evidence is transient and cannot be expected to adhere to other surfaces for very long and it can be dislodged by prolonged contact of the body with the shrouding and bag (Barash *et al.*, 2010).

The clothing of the decedent should be thoroughly examined prior to its removal for autopsy. Furthermore, it is necessary to consider the possibility that clothing might have been removed or added prior to the plant evidence attaching to the clothing (Schierenbeck, 2003; Miller Coyle *et al.*, 2005). Unless the clothing is cut from the victim, the scientist should examine the exposed areas of the skin prior to disrobing the body. Potential evidence can be lost as the clothing is pulled over the hands or feet. In addition, careful examination of the head as well as the body hair may potentially yield plant evidence.

The hands and the feet are excellent sources for plant evidence and should be protected for transport from the scene to the mortuary. The hands (and feet if barefoot) should be covered with unused paper bags and secured around the wrists (and ankles). At autopsy, the bags should be secured as evidence and scrapings should be taken to remove any material from under the nails. The hands and feet should be carefully examined for trace plant material.

When plant evidence is recovered from the autopsy, it is imperative that control samples from the scenes already identified are also obtained. Authorities tasked with this responsibility should be briefed on all aspects regarding the proper collection of plant-related evidence. The plant evidence should be photographed as soon as it is discovered so that its appearance at the time of collection can be documented. Time can alter the appearance of the material so it is critical to observe it in the state in which it was discovered.

Furthermore, it has to be remembered that since much of the value of such evidence comes from possible comparisons, it is necessary to consider potential sources of evidence which can be gathered while the scene is secured and under police control. The environment where a crime occurred can be expected to change over time and the known samples might not be present if too much time has passed between the discovery of plant evidence and the decision to compare it to a known source or reference sample (Miller Coyle, 2005; Laposata, 1985; Barash *et al.*, 2010).

11.6 Laboratory analysis

The basic steps for classification and identification of plant material as forensic evidence are the following: visual assessment, microscopy, chemical and DNA analyses (Miller Coyle, 2005). Each form of testing gives a certain level of information. Visual and microscopic analyses allow for basic classification of pollen or plant material to the species level (Miller Coyle 2005; Hunter, 2006; Schierenbeck, 2003; Miller Coyle *et al.*, 2001, 2005; Brown, 2006; Laposata, 1985; Barash *et al.*, 2010). Chemical and DNA analyses can provide added value by further individualising a sample to the geographic source or original source plant (Miller Coyle *et al.*, 2001, 2005; Mildenhall, 2006a,b; Howard *et al.*, 2009; Craft *et al.*, 2007; Ward *et al.*, 2005).

Plant evidence is submitted to the laboratory for testing in several different formats. Microscopic pollen can be submitted for assessment by scanning electron microscopy (SEM) in sterile vials and is typically collected with sterile paint brushes (Miller Coyle, 2005; see also Chapter 10). Alternatively, tape lifts can be used to easily trap pollen from the scene; however, it can be challenging to remove the pollen from the tape lifts (Miller Coyle, 2005; Barash *et al.*, 2010). The preparation for microscopic analysis should be performed at the laboratory as different forms of microscopy may be used. Due to the miniscule size of pollen grains, SEM is the method of choice to magnify the surface features of the pollen grain which are used to characteristically classify the source of the pollen (Miller Coyle, 2005; Walsh and Horrocks, 2008; Mildenhall *et al.*, 2006). It is rare that sufficient pollen can be collected for effective downstream DNA applications.

For all other forms of plant evidence, the level of characterisation is highly dependent on the type of material collected from the case. A physical match of two plant leaf fragments is a very compelling piece of information. Typically, most criminal cases involve identification of leaves or grass and seeds inadvertently transferred to vehicles, blankets surrounding bodies, shoes or clothing, grave sites or evidence recovered at autopsy (Miller Coyle, 2005; Miller Coyle *et al.*, 2005; Gaensslen *et al.*, 2008; Saferstein, 2009; Girard, 2011; Schierenbeck, 2003). For these circumstances, fresh or wet plant samples can be rubbed on collection cards, air dried and transported to the laboratory for DNA testing (Allgeier *et al.*, 2011). If samples are already dry and brittle, they can be taped flat inside the collection cards and submitted for further microscopic and biological/chemical analysis.

Visual and microscopic analysis of plant fragments involves the photography and descriptive classification of plant material to potential species level using physical features that are present. If the physical features such as vein pattern, leaf shape, colour, striping patterns, textures and thickness are sufficiently unique then identification may be possible. If, however, the physical features are shared by more than one species which is common in some samples such as grasses, then further analyses are necessary. The simplest method for species identification is by DNA (Miller Coyle, 2005; Allgeier *et al.*, 2011; Ferri *et al.*, 2009, 2012; Bruni *et al.*, 2010; Ward *et al.*, 2005, 2009; Howard *et al.*, 2009; Stambuk *et al.*, 2007; Virtanen *et al.*, 2007; Craft *et al.*, 2007; Kress *et al.*, 2005). There are many different genetic loci that are used by evolutionary biologists to classify related plant species (Miller Coyle, 2005; Kress *et al.*, 2005). In forensic botany, this strategy is employed to characterise to the species level plant samples that have similar morphology but are actually derived from separate sources (Ferri *et al.*, 2009, 2012; Bruni *et al.*, 2010; Kress *et al.*, 2005). The best analogy for this is forensic hair analysis. Hair analysis traditionally also involves microscopic assessment for exclusions to a possible source. If the evidentiary sample cannot be excluded, mitochondrial DNA sequencing is performed to characterise the hair to a particular haplotype and include or exclude the sample as being derived from the suspected source such as the victim or the perpetrator (Gaensslen *et al.*, 2008; Saferstein, 2009; Girard, 2011).

Two common sequences used for plant DNA bar-coding are the large subunit of the ribulose-bisphosphate carboxylase gene (rbcL) and the megakaryocyte-associated tyrosine kinase (matK) loci (Kress *et al.*, 2005). These sequences are used to classify a plant sample to the species level by matching sample sequences to known reference sequence information in a public access DNA database (www.ncbi.nlm.nih.gov). Alternatively, a known vouchered reference sample from a herbarium or reliable source can be used as a known reference sample if one is not pre-existent in the NCBI database (Miller Coyle, 2005). Many plant species have short tandem repeat (STR) panels that have been developed for individualisation of a sample and more are being developed all the time. The driving force for the STR panel development is typically for plant breeding strategies by commercial breeders, for patent protection or based on forensic need (Allgeier *et al.*, 2011; Miller Coyle 2001; Ward *et al.*, 2009; Howard *et al.*, 2009; Craft *et al.*, 2007).

11.7 Reporting and court appearance

As with any other specialised area of forensic science, chain of custody documentation and storage conditions of the evidence are of paramount importance (Gaensslen *et al.*, 2008; Saferstein, 2009; Girard, 2011). From the scene to the courtroom, all evidence must be accounted for: where collected, where stored, where tested and where archived.

The integrated and collaborative process of crime scene analysts, forensic scientists, and attorneys requires accurate and complete documentation. Prior to courtroom testimony, the following questions should be addressed (Miller Coyle, 2005):

• Has a review of the evidence from scene, case notes, laboratory notes and signed reports been made? A comprehensive review of the case information by a professional can provide a lot of additional confidence in the value of the plant evidence as well as identify any potential flaws in the methodology used for the case. This review prior to courtroom testimony frequently allows both sides of the case (prosecution and defence) to come to an expedient agreement with a

full understanding of the evidence associated with the case without the expense
of a trial.

- Has plant evidence been previously deemed admissible in your jurisdiction or
  state? If previously admitted by the courts, then a time-consuming and potentially
  costly admissibility hearing is not required. On the one hand, many attorneys are
  wary of trying a case with controversial plant evidence if it will mean an extra
  admissibility hearing. On the other hand, many attorneys would welcome the
  chance to set the benchmark case for court acceptance in their jurisdiction. Plant
  evidence is like any other biological evidence and follows much of the same
  guidelines as are used, for example, for hair analyses. Care in not overstating the
  value of identification at trial testimony is one issue; however, strong scientific
  evidence should not be excluded simply because it has not been routinely used in
  a particular court.

- What are the qualifications of the analysts and specialists in this case? Crime
  scene analysts, law enforcement and evidence technicians are all well qualified
  to collect plant evidence and maintain appropriate documentation and case notes;
  forensic botanists have specialised training in microscopy and DNA testing, and
  all specialists related to the case should meet legal standards for *voir dire* (expert
  credentials) and trial testimony.

- What levels of quality control were used in the collection and testing process?
  The most critical aspects of quality control for plant evidence include appropriate sampling of plant samples for reference at the scene(s), and testing of both
  positive and negative reference controls in conjunction with the evidentiary samples to validate test data at the laboratory. Many laboratories will also include
  blind test samples as a form of quality control during testing. This is analogous
  to proficiency testing of scientists as is standard procedure in all forensic science
  laboratories.

- What is the power of discrimination in the test methods used for this case? Microscopic assessment will necessarily have less power of discrimination than
  DNA testing. This does not invalidate the science but results from some samples
  having common features that do not allow one to distinguish one sample from
  the other by visual examination. The power of discrimination can be increased
  with DNA tests that detect differences in biological molecules from sample to
  sample, just as performed for bloodstains detected at a scene. The types of DNA
  tests that can be performed include DNA sequencing of species markers, STR
  analysis to match samples to reference samples, and single nucleotide poly-
  morphism (SNP) testing to characterise plant samples based on point mutations
  in DNA.

- What are the scientific benefits and limitations to the testing performed? Any
  additional scientific testing that can further associate evidence to a source or
  location is helpful in building a comprehensive knowledge base for the case in

question. As with any scientific test method, care must be taken by the scientist to accurately state the value of the evidence and test results to the court so that appropriate weight can be given to the evidence.

11.8 Conclusion

Forensic botany is a unique evidential aspect at a crime scene that is often overlooked due to lack of knowledge regarding its potential. Many crime scene analysts do not know that plant evidence can be evaluated like many other types of trace materials at sophisticated chemical and biological levels. Most forensic science laboratories do not have a forensic botanist on staff; however, a handful of qualified forensic botanists perform consulting and training across the United States and worldwide on request. Training for plant evidence collection on collection cards can aid in preserving the chemical and biological substances necessary for more sophisticated analyses to not only classify botanical evidence to the species level but to use DNA and chemistry to individualise that sample to a source plant. Crime scene analysts or investigators need to be aware that reference samples and reference populations from the geographic area surrounding the crime scene will need to be collected for comparison to the evidentiary materials too and could be transient in nature. In addition, instead of storing trace plant material in dry coin envelopes, sending the collection cards out to qualified laboratories for immediate analysis is beneficial to the case.

All plants contain characteristic combinations of chemicals that can aid in classification. DNA, in particular, can be used to confirm a species using highly conserved DNA sequences such as the rbcL or trnA genes. This form of information can be checked against a database for quick comparisons and reports back to crime scene analysts for investigative leads. This technology has been available in the research community for years but has never been systematically installed for use by forensic scientists and crime scene investigators in the legal arena.

Finally, proper collection guidelines for crime scenes and bodies with associated botanical evidence have been presented here as a reference. Greater use of plant bioinformatics databases are a vision for the future where all the biological evidence, including pollen, food, and trace plants and drugs will be assessed at the crime scene and rapidly collected and analysed on-site or sent for immediate analysis at the forensic science laboratory to aid in case resolution.

References

Allgeier, L., Hemenway, J., Shirley, N. *et al*. 2011. Field testing of collection cards for *Cannabis sativa* samples with a single hexanucleotide DNA marker. *Journal of Forensic Sciences* **56**: 1245–1249.

Barash, M., Reshef, A. and Brauner, P. 2010. The use of adhesive tape for recovery of DNA from crime scene items. *Journal of Forensic Sciences* **55**: 1058–1064.

Brown, A.G. 2006. The use of forensic botany and geology in war crimes investigations in NE Bosnia. *Forensic Science International* **163**: 204–210.

Bruni, I., De Mattia, F., Galimberti, A. *et al.* 2010. Identification of poisonous plants by DNA barcoding approach. *International Journal of Legal Medicine* **124**: 595–603.

Craft, K.J., Owens, J.D. and Ashley, M.V. 2007. Application of plant DNA markers in forensic botany: genetic comparison of *Quercus* evidence leaves to crime scene trees using microsatellites. *Forensic Science International* **165**: 64–70.

Ferri, G., Corradini, B. and Alù, M. 2012. Capillary electrophoresis of multigene barcoding chloroplast markers for species identification of botanical trace evidence. *Methods in Molecular Biology* **830**: 253–263.

Ferri, G., Alù, M., Corradini, B. and Beduschi, G. 2009. Forensic botany: species identification of botanical trace evidence using a multigene barcoding approach. *International Journal of Legal Medicine* **123**: 395–401.

Gaensslen, R., Harris, H. and Lee, H. (eds) 2008. *Introduction to Forensic Science & Criminalistics*. McGraw-Hill, New York, NY.

Girard, J. (ed.) 2011. *Criminalistics: Forensic Science, Crime, and Terrorism*. Jones & Bartlett Learning LLC, Sudbury, MA.

Howard, C., Gilmore, S., Robertson, J. and Peakall, R. 2009. A *Cannabis sativa* STR genotype database for Australian seizures: forensic applications and limitations. *Journal of Forensic Sciences* **54**: 556–563.

Hunter, P. 2006. All the evidence. *EMBO Reports* **7**: 352–354.

Kress, W.J., Wurdack, K.J., Zimmer, E.A. *et al.* 2005. Use of DNA barcodes to identify flowering plants. *Proceedings of the National Academy of Sciences* **102**: 8369–8374.

Laposata, E.A. 1985. Collection of trace evidence from bombing victims at autopsy. *Journal of Forensic Sciences* **30**: 789–797.

Mildenhall, D.C. 2006a. An unusual appearance of a common pollen type indicates the scene of the crime. *Forensic Science International* **163**: 236–240.

Mildenhall, D.C. 2006b. *Hypericum* pollen determines the presence of burglars at the scene of a crime: an example of forensic palynology. *Forensic Science International* **163**: 231–235.

Mildenhall, D.C., Wiltshire, P.E. and Bryant, V.M. 2006. Forensic palynology: why do it and how it works. *Forensic Science International* **163**: 163–172.

Miller Coyle, H. (ed.) 2005. *Forensic Botany: Principles and Applications to Criminal Casework*. CRC Press, Boca Raton, FL.

Miller Coyle, H., Ladd, C., Palmbach, T. and Lee, H.C. 2001. The Green Revolution: botanical contributions to forensics and drug enforcement. *Croatian Medical Journal* **42**: 340–345.

Miller Coyle, H., Lee, C.L., Lin, W.Y. *et al.* 2005. Forensic botany: using plant evidence to aid in forensic death investigation. *Croatian Medical Journal* **46**: 606–612.

Saferstein, R. (ed.) 2009. *Forensic Science: From the Crime Scene to the Crime Lab*. Pearson Education Inc., Upper Saddle River, NJ.

Schierenbeck, K.A. 2003. Forensic biology. *Journal of Forensic Sciences* **48**: 696.

Stambuk, S., Sutlović, D., Bakarić, P. *et al.* 2007. Forensic botany: potential usefulness of microsatellite-based genotyping of Croatian olive (*Olea europaea* L.) in forensic casework. *Croatian Medical Journal* **48**: 556–562.

Virtanen, V., Korpelainen, H. and Kostamo, K. 2007. Forensic botany: usability of bryophyte material in forensic studies. *Forensic Science International* **172**: 161–163.

Walsh, K.A. and Horrocks, M. 2008. Palynology: its position in the field of forensic science. *Journal of Forensic Sciences* **53**: 1053–1060.

Ward, J., Gilmore, S.R., Robertson, J. and Peakall, R. 2009. A grass molecular identification system for forensic botany: a critical evaluation of the strengths and limitations. *Journal of Forensic Sciences* **54**: 1254–1260.

Ward, J., Peakall, R., Gilmore, S.R. and Robertson, J. 2005. A molecular identification system for grasses: a novel technology for forensic botany. *Forensic Science International* **152**: 121–131.

Wu, C-L., Yang, C-H., Huang, T-C. and Chen, S-H. 2006. Forensic pollen evidence from clothes by the tape adhesive method. *Taiwania* **51**: 123–130.

12

Forensic geology and soils

Duncan Pirrie[1] and Alastair Ruffell[2]
[1] Helford Geoscience LLP, Penryn, UK
[2] School of Geography, Archaeology and Palaeoecology, Queen's University Belfast, Belfast, UK

12.1 Introduction and current state of the discipline

Forensic geology (also referred to as geoforensics or forensic geoscience) is the scientific study of geological materials, or the use of geological scientific techniques, in a forensic context. Typically, there are two separate, but commonly complementary subdisciplines: search and trace evidence. With search, background geological knowledge and a range of instrumental and analytical techniques can be deployed in the search for objects either on the land surface, buried, disposed of in water, or subsurface voids (naturally occurring caves, but also man-made structures such as mines, shafts and drainage adits). Geological trace evidence includes rocks, sediments and dusts, but most commonly in a forensic context, involves the analysis and comparison of soil samples. Less commonly, it also includes man-made substances like concrete and mineral products (e.g. plaster). Geological trace evidence has been utilised repeatedly in serious criminal investigations, not only in the United Kingdom, but worldwide. Its uptake and acceptance by investigating officers has varied considerably over the last 10–20 years, but at present (as the result of a range of initiatives), there has been an increase in the use of soils and other classes of geological trace evidence in serious crime investigations. In the United Kingdom, the establishment of a specialist group of the Geological Society of London – *the Forensic Geoscience Group* – has promoted the use of geoscience in forensic investigations and has also led to a series of scientific conferences. Possibly more significant has been the establishment in 2011, of the International Union of Geological Sciences (IUGS) Initiative on Forensic Geology. This project has brought together practising forensic geoscientists from around the world (e.g. UK, France, Germany, Italy, Portugal, Russia, USA, Australia, New Zealand, South Africa, UAE, Brazil, Colombia, etc.) along with international law enforcement agencies, and an early aim of the Initiative is to publish a '*Guide to Forensic Geology*' by bringing together this

Forensic Ecology Handbook: From Crime Scene to Court, First Edition.
Edited by Nicholas Márquez-Grant and Julie Roberts.
© 2012 John Wiley & Sons, Ltd. Published 2012 by John Wiley & Sons, Ltd.

international expertise. This will help in the development of best practice protocols and standard operating procedures which can then be adapted to make them appropriate for the investigative and legal frameworks operating in different countries around the world. Whilst geologists are becoming more aware of the value of their subject in forensic investigations, this is not always the case with senior investigating officers (SIOs), crime scene managers (CSMs) or crime scene investigators (CSIs), as well as other law enforcement personnel, such as those investigating environmental or wildlife crime. Soils are not just soils, rocks are not just rocks, and the aim of this chapter is to explain how they can form important classes of trace evidence in police investigations. A brief overview of the ways in which geology can aid in search is presented, but the primary aim of this contribution is to consider geological trace evidence.

12.1.1   Why is geological trace evidence of value?

If one thinks about the United Kingdom, there is a huge range in landscapes, from the chalk downs of southern England to the granite moors of Devon and Cornwall. The richness of the UK landscape (which in turn strongly influences its flora) is due to the diversity of our underlying geology. For a country with such a relatively small area, we have an extremely diverse and variable underlying geology. If one was to take a cross-section through the surface of the land in most parts of the United Kingdom, one would encounter the surface and subsurface soils; these commonly overlie superficial or drift deposits of fluvial, lacustrine, glacial or periglacial origin and then the underlying solid bedrock. Within the near-surface soils and commonly subsoils, there will be the addition of man-made materials, even in rural settings. Together all of these materials make surface and subsurface rocks and soils very variable, and it is this variability that allows geological analysis of value in a forensic investigation. The scientifically recognised variability of soils, however, often goes hand in hand with a perception amongst the general public that soil is just soil. Thus whilst offenders may recognise that DNA might link them to a crime scene, there is much less understanding that a soil sample from an item of footwear might also link the offender to the scene. Sadly, that misunderstanding is also commonplace with SIOs and CSIs.

There is also a common misunderstanding that soil or geological trace evidence only has value if the crime scene is in a rural location, such as the disposal of a body in a shallow grave, or the surface deposition of a victim in woodland. Many urban environments are very variable and very complex and therefore have considerable potential for trace evidence. For example, in many city centres in the United Kingdom there are brownfield sites awaiting redevelopment. Such past industrial sites are frequently used for the legal and illegal tipping of wastes, and with each new material being added to a site its distinctiveness increases. They are also relatively common scenes for the disposal of bodies. Thus geological and soil trace evidence has an equally important role in an urban scene as in a rural scene.

The most commonly encountered materials in forensic geology investigations are soils and sediments, as it is these surface and near-surface materials that offenders and victims are likely to come into contact with. Soils are complex mixtures of natural inorganic particles (minerals), organic components (e.g. macroscopic plant fragments, pollen, spores) and man-made materials. As such there is commonly a strong overlap between forensic geology and forensic palynology/forensic botany. It can be viewed that the minerals and the palynomorphs present in a single soil sample are two different classes of trace evidence that are present in the same matrix. Thus, if both classes of trace evidence are examined by independent experts then they can provide complementary evidence when a case comes to court. In most serious criminal investigations it would be best practice to have both a forensic geologist and a forensic palynologist/botanist examining the same soil samples. This may not, however, be possible, if, for example, the critical exhibits (e.g. from an item of footwear) are too small for both disciplines to have appropriate samples for analysis. In this case, one or other approach would need to be selected based on the nature of the case. For instance, if the scene was rural, heavily vegetated with little in the way of exposed soils then a forensic palynology/botany approach may be more appropriate; if the site was a poorly vegetated area of waste ground with dumped construction wastes, then a geological approach may be more suitable. These are of course extreme examples, and in many cases which approach to follow may not be so clear-cut. Unfortunately, there are no data to suggest in advance of carrying out the work for a specific case, whether the geological components or the biological components of a soil will provide the strongest evidential value.

12.1.2 Role of geological techniques in search

In some cases, there may be a requirement to try to identify areas where an object may have been hidden. Typically this may be in a missing murder victim enquiry. Geological assistance can be of value in helping to define or narrow down search parameters, even in the absence of any available trace evidence. Let us first consider the case where there is trace evidence from a possible offender (e.g. item of footwear; digging implement; soil on a motor vehicle) but the location where that trace evidence may have come from is unknown. In this scenario, detailed geological and botanical (potentially also entomological and other evidence types) examination and analysis of the exhibits would be warranted. Commonly such analysis can allow large areas of land to be excluded from consideration as the soils could simply not have been derived from those locations. By excluding areas, this can allow more focused consideration on smaller areas of potential interest. Rarely will the combined trace evidence allow the definition of a discrete place; instead the data will describe the nature of that place, the underlying soils and geology, proximity to industrial activity, nature of vegetation, proximity to water, etc. These data then need to be combined with other strands of evidence to try to localise the search area(s). Very infrequently, a rare combination of materials may be present in a soil sample so that a discrete place can be identified, but usually there is an insufficient database to enable an individual location to be identified.

A more complex situation would be the search for a clandestine grave, when there is no trace evidence to indicate the location and only broad intelligence to suggest the possible areas. Initial contact between the investigating officer and a geologist should not be a field visit where the former presumes the latter will magically conjure up a burial location. Instead, a full desktop study of the search area needs to be conducted. This will include all available information on geology, soils, topography and hydrology, past land use (from old OS maps, verbal accounts from local inhabitants), and current land use (from satellite and aerial imagery). This desk-based assessment is invaluable as it may prevent some nasty surprises, such as finding building works where none were anticipated, or preventing the search team from falling into a bog! At an early stage an assessment of the underlying geology can be significant in predicting the diggability of the ground – that is, the ease with which a clandestine grave could be prepared. This can be compared with surface elevation data and groundwater conditions amongst others to identify areas which can effectively be excluded from consideration based on the predictable ground conditions. Note as well that many areas of the world have had a long mining history and in many areas, there are abandoned mines and quarries which can provide easy localities for the disposal of victims of homicide, as well as accidental deaths, or other buried objects. Such sites can be easily assessed by a geologist but may be less obvious to a non-specialist. Once small-scale targets have been located then there is a wide array of instruments available which can be deployed to help in the search for areas of ground disturbance. Such techniques fall at the boundary between forensic geology, near-surface geophysics and forensic archaeology. At the present time in the United Kingdom and elsewhere there are a number of companies and universities with capability and active programmes of research into instrumentation for the search for ground disturbances on land and also the disposal of objects in bodies of water. Whilst many will be aware of techniques such as the use of ground penetrating radar, the selection of the instruments to be used is fundamentally controlled by the likely ground conditions that will be encountered at a specific search location and need to be tailored accordingly if the search is to have value. These techniques are, however, beyond the scope of this contribution.

12.2 Applications for forensic geology

There are a number of different areas in which forensic geoscience might aid an enquiry:

1. *Rocks and ceramics (e.g. bricks) as weapons, or in the disposal of objects in water.* Where rocks or man-made materials such as bricks have been used as weapons, geological input can provide information on the source of that material. For example, in one case an individual had been repeatedly struck with a rock,

whilst standing at or just inside the doorway of their home address. The question posed was: Had the rock been picked up within the victim's garden or had it been brought to the place of the offence? Another example was whether or not rocks thrown through a victim's window were similar to rock samples found at a suspect's home address. Other enquiries have regarded identifying where rock samples used to weigh down bags dumped in standing bodies of water were potentially sourced from. In addition to rocks, man-made construction materials such as bricks and concrete are also distinctive and their source (origin) can be identified.

2. *Geological trace evidence linking a suspect or victim to a scene.* This is the most common area where geological trace evidence has been used. Typically this will involve the recovery of geological trace evidence from, for example, a vehicle, items of footwear or clothing, or other implements (the questioned samples), and the comparison of these exhibits with samples collected from both the crime scene and also from other relevant comparator locations (the crime scene and control samples). Some practitioners prefer to call this 'the exclusionary method' whereby all possible alibi location are discounted until only the questioned sample and crime scene are left to be compared. Soil trace evidence is most commonly used in murder enquiries, and usually when other forensic avenues have proven unsuccessful. Soil sampling should, however, be part of the standard forensic protocol at such scenes (see Section 12.4).

3. *Geological trace evidence to identify unknown locations.* Geological trace evidence can also be utilised to describe the nature of unknown places based on the recovery and analysis of materials from exhibits. This can be used in, for example, the search for missing murder victims; but it can also be used in identifying the movements of materials. With missing victim murder enquiries a significant amount of resources can be deployed to try to locate potential target search areas. Making use of any available trace evidence from suspects at this stage can be very cost-effective in terms of localising the search area. However, we have previously been told that a CSM would only allow the analysis of the trace evidence from an exhibit once the body deposition sight was located and could not grasp the idea that the trace evidence might actually lead the search to the body deposition site. Geological particles can easily become attached to packaging materials, and if recovered and analysed appropriately, can be used to identify the sources of those particles. Such 'geolocation' studies can be carried out on a global level. A case we worked on involved the substitution of high-value experimental computer drives. These were manufactured in Taiwan and air-freighted via Budapest (Hungary) and Gatwick (southern England) to their destination near Londonderry (Northern Ireland). Upon arrival, the parts had been substituted for some bags of soil, some roofing tiles and rocks. The question was: Where had the substitution taken place? As described above, a conjunctive approach, using both geological and palynological (pollen, see Chapter 10) analysis was undertaken. The rocks were of a kind known as flysch – common in Alpine terrains; the pollens were of a Mediterranean type, the roof tiles likewise of a Mediterranean

type. These independent lines of evidence excluded Taiwan, England and Northern Ireland, but could be accounted for by a switch being made in Hungary. Enquiries at Budapest Airport led to the confession of a suspect. Commonly, such 'geolocation' studies can enable large areas to be excluded and then provide a description of the nature of the place(s) the particles may have been sourced from, as in the case above. In addition, man-made particulates can also provide an indication of the types of activities being carried out.

4. *Geological trace evidence in fatal road traffic incidents.* Recently we have carried out casework for a number of investigations into fatal road traffic incidents. In one case, where a car driver died after having rocks thrown at the vehicle/road carriageway from a bridge, it was possible to link trace evidence from the rocks recovered from the carriageway with trace evidence from the pockets of an item of clothing belonging to a suspect. It appeared that the suspect had filled their pockets with rocks before going on to the bridge as there was no available source for projectiles actually up on the bridge. In a separate case of a fatal road traffic collision the question posed related to where mud on a carriageway had come from, which had resulted in a driver losing control of their vehicle.

5. *Stolen geological materials.* The direct theft of geological materials is a relatively rare offence in the United Kingdom, but cases include the theft of roofing slates, roofing tiles and other materials. Forensic geology can aid in the identification of the likely provenance of seized, suspected stolen materials. This type of work is of far greater significance in other areas of the world, such as South Africa, where high value geological commodities (e.g. gold, platinum) can be stolen, shipped around the world and then sold back into the supply chain. Just as soil is not just soil; gold, silver, rare metals and gems all have unique properties and can be analysed to track their source.

In *our* opinion, there are, however, a range of offences where soil trace evidence has been under-utilised in both serious crimes and also less serious volume crimes. For example, it is not uncommon for sexual assaults (e.g. rapes) to occur in parks, alleyways and areas of waste ground. Both the victim and the offender may easily contact the ground surface. The distribution of geological trace evidence on a victim and an offender's clothing and footwear could be used to independently test different scenarios. Whilst used in some cases, it has rarely been used, possibly due to an over-reliance on more traditional forensic approaches.

At the present time, high scrap metal prices have led to a significant increase in the theft of metal. In some cases, such as the theft of cables from railway lines, there is both the financial cost, but also a considerable cost in terms of the disruption to the rail network, and also the potential risk to life for those involved in such offences. Offenders have to contact trackside locations, which will be characterised by not only the geological materials used as the rail ballast, but also the local soils and other particulates. Given that these track-side locations are not publicly accessible there is no legitimate reason for individuals to have trace evidence on their clothing for example, from such locations. It may also be possible through detailed analysis of recovered metals, that the source of those metals can be identified. Other volume crimes such as burglary are also potential areas where forensic geoscience may play a role in the conviction of offenders as commonly individuals may be in contact with soils in a victim's garden. The under-utilisation of geological trace evidence is probably because of: (a) a lack of awareness of the potential; and (b) a view that such specialist work is too costly.

12.3   Pre-scene attendance

As with all forensic disciplines, early involvement is commonly highly beneficial to the end result. Although as discussed below in Section 12.4, we do not consider that this automatically means that scene attendance will be required. At the outset, the SIO, CSM or CSI needs to consider whether geological trace evidence may have a potential role in the investigation. Clearly this does not have to be a priority in terms of analysis as more mainstream forensic strategies can be carried out in advance, but at the outset, it is recommended that consideration is given as to whether geology may have value.

The pre-scene preparation really depends on the nature of the case. In all cases the forensic geologist needs to be briefed as thoroughly as possible, so that they can make a recommendation as to whether or not geology may aid the enquiry. If this is the recommendation then a forensic strategy can be prepared. To do this the forensic geologist needs information: (a) what is the nature of the offence and when did it occur; (b) when were critical exhibits (e.g. footwear etc.) seized; (c) what are the critical questions that the investigative team want to test; (d) where is the offence though to have occurred; and (e) what were the weather conditions at the time of the offence.

At some relatively simple scenes there may be no requirement for a forensic geologist to attend; sampling can be carried out by a suitably trained CSI. At complex scenes, attendance by a forensic geologist may be required. To assess whether or not a specialist is required on scene can be easily achieved by sending the specialist digital photographs (see Chapter 14) of the scene for evaluation; although it should be borne in mind that a specialist sees the world differently to a non-specialist. Aspects of pre-scene preparation which can be carried out by a geologist are:

(a) an assessment of the terrain and landscape;

(b) an assessment of the underlying bedrock geology;

(c) a consideration (based on the nature of the offence) about the best sampling strategy to be utilised and what equipment will be required.

Commonly, soil sampling is often considered after the 'event' when other forensic strategies have not assisted; this is not ideal and sampling should be carried out at the time of the initial investigation. However, if sampling is being carried out retrospectively then the same level of support should be put in place: for instance attendance of a CSI along with the forensic geologist, a police photographer and a crime scene mapper. A competent forensic geologist is perfectly capable of locating sampling locations, photographing the sampling locations and recovering and packaging the exhibits, but best practice would ensure that support staff are in attendance.

12.4 Scene attendance and sampling

The whole premise behind soil sampling for forensic geology is that soils are very variable materials, and this has to be foremost in the mind when sampling is carried out to ensure that appropriate samples are collected. The specific details of the case will control whether or not a forensic geologist is required at the scene, or whether sampling can be carried out by a CSI. It may be possible to send scene photographs to a forensic geologist to enable them to advise on whether or not their attendance is required and if not, on the best sampling strategy to be adopted. Sampling of soils is clearly not the highest priority, but should be carried out as early on as possible.

12.4.1 Soil sampling at a surface body deposition site

With a scenario where a body is discovered deposited on a ground surface, the sampling strategy needs to focus on those surfaces where an offender would have contacted any soils. How was the body moved to the scene? Would the offender have only been standing or is there any indication that they may have knelt down? Can the approach path to the body deposition site be identified? If the approach path can be identified then soil samples should be collected around the body (head, feet, left and right side of the body) (Figure 12.1a). Samples should then be collected along the approach path and also in any areas where, for example, an offender may have parked a vehicle (Figure 12.1b). In this scenario detailed targeted sampling is required in the exact areas where an offender may have contacted the surface. If there are discrete footwear marks present then soil samples can be recovered following the casting of the marks, although a subsample of the casting agents should also be retained as they may cross-contaminate the soil samples (Figure 12.1c). Sampling needs to focus on the surfaces that the offender may have contacted; clearly the exact location where each soil sample is to be collected from needs to be accurately surveyed, and the area photographed before samples are recovered. In the absence of footwear marks, it is recommended that a 20×20 cm area is sampled by gently scraping the surface using a sterile spatula. The depth of the sample depends on how wet the soils are and effectively it is necessary to sample down to the depth to which the tread of an item of footwear would go to. In other words, if the surface is dry then the sampling depth would be the uppermost mm or two; if the soils are

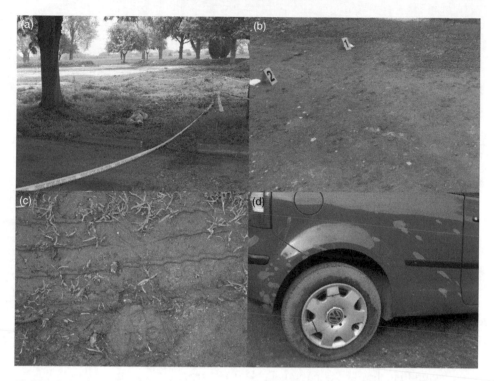

Figure 12.1 Soil sampling in forensic geology investigations. (a) With a surface body deposition, soil samples should be collected around the victim, taking into account the likely way in which the body was moved by the offender(s). In this case samples would also be taken from the adjacent road. Image courtesy of Manlove Forensics training course. (b) Areas such as this loosely surfaced car park can be very distinctive geologically because of the mix of both naturally occurring soils and introduced materials such as aggregates. (c) Where there are distinct vehicle tracks or footwear impressions, soil samples can either be taken from the impression itself or from a cast of the impression. (d) When sampling vehicles and other exhibits, the primary aim is to identify discrete depositional events; in this case the obvious mud splashes on the bodywork of a vehicle. (To see a colour version of this figure, please see Plate 12.1.)

wet and muddy then sampling down to 1cm would be appropriate. Sampling depth is important as soil characteristics can vary with depth, even on a millimetre scale. Samples should be collected along the length of the offender approach path. If this leads to an area where a vehicle may have been parked then samples should also be targeted around where a vehicle may have been and where an offender may have stood whilst getting into, or out of, a vehicle (Figure 12.1a).

In this scenario if the scene was rural and all of the soils in the area appeared the same with regard to colour and texture, then a forensic geologist may not be required at the scene and sampling can be carried out as part of the overall strategy by the CSI. However, if the body was deposited in an area where there are obvious visual differences in the soil types present, then the sampling strategy will be more complex, requiring all soil types to be sampled, and attendance at the scene by a specialist would be recommended.

The scene sampling procedure is therefore:

1. Identify areas where an offender may have contacted the ground surface.

2. Target sampling to these specific areas and survey in the locations at which soil samples are to be recovered.

3. Photograph the sampling locations prior to sampling.

4. Collect soil samples by gently scraping across the surface of the soils in an area of approximately 20 by 20 cm and to a depth as indicated by the soil conditions (surface mm if dry; down to a depth of ~1cm if wet and muddy). Sampling can be carried out using a sterile spatula or similar. Either clean the sampling instrument thoroughly between each sample location, or use a new one. Do not cross-contaminate the different samples. Sampling can be most easily achieved by scraping the surface soils onto a piece of paper which can then be sealed in an evidence bag.

5. Target sampling to areas around the victim's body and along the likely offender approach path. The number of samples to be collected depends on the complexity of the scene; more is better than less – they may not all be examined, but once collected then they are at least available if required.

Finally, soil sampling should be carried out at the time of the body recovery; soil compositions can change with time (particularly the palynology) hence although samples could be collected at a later stage they may no longer be representative of the soils at the time of the offence. Sometimes the ground is dry and dusty, making sampling with a spatula problematic, as scraping tends to flick the particles around. An alternative is to use a new toothbrush and piece of paper and gently brush the appropriate surface (usually with dusty material a few millimetres) onto the paper, to be folded, labelled and sealed in an evidence bag with the same unique name/number. A new toothbrush must be used for each sample and if possible, place the used toothbrush itself in the evidence bag since the bristles often capture a remarkable amount of debris.

12.4.2 Soil sampling at a shallow burial

The strategy to be adopted at a burial is the same as a surface deposition, except that soils from the grave fill also need to be sampled. Soil characteristics vary with depth such that when a grave is dug and then backfilled, typically the soils from different depths will be mixed. This can be of considerable value in a forensic context as if the offender has contacted the soils placed within the grave, then the soils will be distinctive of the grave fill itself rather than just the general deposition site. Soil samples need to be collected from the surface of the grave fill, prior to excavation, and then from deeper in the grave fill itself. Finally, a soil sample should also be taken from the base of the grave cut, in case the offender has stood inside the grave itself. Otherwise, a burial location should be dealt with from a sampling strategy in the same way as for a surface body deposition site.

12.4.3 Geological trace evidence recovery from vehicles

The recovery of geological trace evidence from vehicles should be carried out by a forensic geologist, potentially as part of a joint examination by other forensic specialists (e.g. examining for the presence of blood). This is particularly important in missing person murder enquiries where a vehicle is suspected of having been used in the transfer of a victim. Historically the types of samples recovered from vehicles have included sweepings from foot-wells and scrapings from wheel arches, but in our experience other samples to target include mud splashes all over the vehicle, debris on the foot pedals and from items placed in the boot. Usually such samples have no forensic value as they will be mixed samples, representing all of the places visited by the vehicles and any passengers travelling in it. With advances in analytical techniques, it is possible to gain significant information from smaller and smaller samples, and as such the examination and sampling of a vehicle needs to focus on the recovery of soils representative of discrete depositional events and places (Figure 12.1d). For example, if a person gets into a vehicle with muddy footwear and scuffs the door panel trim, then this discrete soil sample is representative of the place that soil was derived from. During the examination and sampling of a vehicle, care needs to be exercised to minimise cross-contamination between different parts of the vehicle and the environment in which the vehicle is being stored. Forensic garages are rarely clean environments, and ideally the vehicle should be protected from the garage surface using plastic or paper.

The exterior of the vehicle can be systematically examined and any discrete areas of soil can be described, photographed and then sampled. Any clods of soil on the bodywork (Figure 12.1d) can be removed using a scalpel or spatula and packaged separately. Sampling of wheel arches depends on the time period between the alleged offence and when the vehicle was seized. If a significant period of time has elapsed, and the vehicle is known to have been used in the intervening period, then there is little value to be gained from sampling the wheel arches. If, however, the vehicle has been seized within a few days of the offence, then the uppermost layer of soils within the wheel arch should be sampled. Theoretically, soils within a wheel arch build up through a series of successive depositional events, and it may in future prove possible to recover micro-cores through the soil build-ups, in an attempt to identify discrete places. For a detailed vehicle examination, an inspection pit or ramp is required so that the underside of the vehicle can also be examined; soils can be retained on the underside of a vehicle, on, for example, the suspension arm struts, for considerable periods of time. In addition, examination should also be carried out within the engine compartment, as leaves, for example, can become lodged under the vehicle bonnet. Stones lodged within the tyre tread should also be removed and retained as separate exhibits; they may just be from commonly used road aggregates or they may come from loose aggregates on the surface of a track-way or car park area. If there are discrete areas of soil on the side-walls of the tyres then they should also be recovered. Note again that it is essential that during the sampling there is no cross-contamination of the different soils present.

Once the exterior of the vehicle has been examined and sampled, then the interior can be examined. Ideally this should be done without entering the vehicle although in some case (e.g. examination of large vans) this will not be possible, in which case care needs to be exercised to ensure that the vehicle is not cross-contaminated by particulate debris from the surface of the forensic garage. Once again, the interior needs to be examined for discrete soil depositional events: examine door panels, car mats, carpets, etc. It will also be necessary to look inside door pockets (muddy items may have been placed inside them and soils may be present). In many cases it may be best to remove items with any soils *in situ* so that they can be examined and recovered under laboratory conditions. For example, areas of trim with adhering soils can be cut out and packaged; car mats and carpets can be removed and packaged as separate exhibits. The vehicle clutch, brake and accelerator pedals can usually be removed intact and can be packaged as separate exhibits. If, however, there are loose clods of soils, or small rock fragments present, then they should be photographed *in situ* and then removed (e.g. using tweezers and secured in an evidence container).

The *in situ* sweeping of foot-wells will generally result in a sample that reflects numerous different places, hence is of little value. In such cases it is better that the car mats are removed intact and then packaged for laboratory examination, rather than being sampled within a forensic garage. If sweeping samples have to be taken, then one must ensure that a different brush is used for each foot-well; otherwise the samples will be cross-contaminated. Finally, if the weather conditions, scene security, etc. permit, it is worth considering treating vehicles as discrete scenes, and carrying out an examination and sampling at the scene where the vehicle is seized rather than transporting it to a forensic garage where cross-contamination may be an issue.

12.4.4 Comparator (or control) samples

Typically in most forensic geoscience investigations, one may have a suite of samples collected from a crime scene along with a suite of samples collected from exhibits seized from individual(s) of interest to the enquiry. The two suites of samples can be analysed to test the hypothesis that the soil samples present on the exhibits were derived through contact with exposed soils present at the crime scene. However, additional comparator or control samples should also be collected for analysis. These might include: (1) additional samples from the area around the crime scene to evaluate the spatial variability in soil compositions in that area; and (2) the collection of soil samples from locations where the individuals of interest to the enquiry might have come into contact with soils, sometimes referred to as alibi locations. This might include their home addresses, places of work, and also places where they might carry out recreation. With increasing pressure on police budgets getting authorisation for such sampling is commonly seen as something of a luxury, but it is very important in the evaluation of the evidential significance of the findings.

12.5 Sampling and preparation in the laboratory

Once exhibits have been seized or recovered then they can be submitted to an appropriate laboratory for examination. As geological trace evidence commonly is complementary to forensic botany (see Chapter 11) or palynology (see Chapter 10), examination and sampling should be carried out in such a way that there is no potential risk of cross-contamination and also so that samples are also recovered for these other disciplines. Clearly, exhibits must be examined under appropriate clean laboratory facilities and using full PPE (personal protective equipment). Laboratories should ideally have a positive airflow system, ensuring that there is no cross-contamination with airborne spores and pollen. The sequence and locations in which different exhibits should be examined must be carefully considered, to ensure that there is no possibility of cross-contamination. All exhibit examinations must be clearly and fully documented and no samples should be recovered before the exhibits are fully photographed showing the trace evidence in context with the exhibits.

12.5.1 Geological trace evidence recovery from footwear, clothing, etc.

The recovery of geological trace evidence from exhibits such as clothing, footwear and digging implements should be carried out by the forensic geologist under laboratory conditions. Examination can be carried out visually and using microscopy, before sample recovery. Detailed sampling can be carried out, enabling subsamples to be collected for both geological and palynological/botanical analysis. If sampling has to be carried out by a non-specialist, then it is recommended that items are digitally photographed and advice on sampling is sought from an appropriate expert before sampling is carried out. Again, the forensic sampling strategy is to try to ensure that individual soil samples representing discrete places are recovered separately. If exhibits have been stored appropriately, then soils can still be recovered from items from cold cases; there have been very significant advances in analytical techniques which today mean that smaller samples can be utilised. During cold case reviews these advances should be borne in mind; the examination of old exhibits can still yield valuable evidence in an investigation. We carried out analyses on a pair of jeans worn by a murder victim that had been stored for 15 years. The adhered mud could still be analysed for mineralogy, and contained the remains of (dead) microscopic organisms known as testate amoebae. These results allowed us to exclude one possible murder location (the site of the abduction of the victim) and include the body deposition site as the likely murder scene. This information was later used in a reconstruction for the UK television programme *Crimewatch*.

12.5.2 Geological trace evidence recovery from victims and suspects

It is relatively rare to recover trace geological evidence from the skin, hair or nostrils of a victim or suspect, but it can be done in some circumstances. Examples of situations where this may be required would be, for example, when a naked body is recovered and there are soils, sediments or macroscopic vegetation present on the surface of the skin or in the victim's hair. Do those soils relate to the body deposition site or some other location? This may be of importance in bodies recovered from rivers: Does soil or sediment on the body come from the river, or a location along the river bank where they entered the water?

Soil samples can be recovered by washing the skin or hair and catching the washings in a sterile container; the washing sample can then be placed into a suitable container and frozen. Soil or sediment samples may also be recovered from under the finger nails: in one of our recent cases, the pathologist suggested that a murder victim may have clawed at the ground with her hands in an attempt to escape her assailant. We were able to exclude the mud under her fingernails from the body deposition site, and unless the victim had dirty nails in life, this result could suggest another location for the attack.

12.5.3 Sample storage

There are differing opinions as to the best options for long-term sample storage. Some palynologists and botanists recommend that soil samples are stored frozen, although others have argued that freezing may affect some attributes of the soils. In general, the simplest recommendation is that soil samples should be stored dry. When samples are collected either damp or wet, then they should be dried prior to storage. Drying in a drying cabinet at temperatures of up to 50°C is unlikely to detrimentally affect the sample in any way, although care needs to be exercised to ensure that the samples are not cross-contaminated. Sample packaging also needs to be carefully considered. Ideally, dry soils should be folded up within a piece of paper which can then be sealed within a zip-lock plastic bag and then within a plastic or paper evidence bag. Soil samples should not be placed within petri dishes as they can easily leak; even if sealed with tape it is common for particles to end up adhering to the sealing tape. Small samples can be placed within Eppendorf tubes or similar storage tubes.

12.6 Laboratory analysis

At the present time there is no standardised analytical protocol for the examination of geological trace evidence. It is hoped that the IUGS Initiative on Forensic Geology (see Section 12.1) will provide recommendations in due course, although the methods adopted will depend on the expertise of the individual forensic geologist and the availability of analytical equipment. The reason why there is no standardised approach to the forensic analysis of geological trace evidence is because there are many different parameters which can be measured. If we initially consider a soil or sediment sample, then we can either examine the overall bulk composition of that sample, or we can examine the characteristics of individual particles making up that sample. The wide range of different analytical techniques are discussed at length in recently published textbooks and volumes arising from forensic geology conferences as well as papers published in international forensic science journals (e.g. Murray, 2004; Pye and Croft, 2004; Pye, 2007; Ruffell and McKinley, 2008; Ritz, Dawson and Miller, 2009). Consequently the wide range of analytical methods is not considered in detail here; the specific analytical approach adopted will depend on the nature of the particular case and the expert witness appointed. However, it is worth considering the types of information that can be gleaned through different analytical techniques.

In general most laboratories will work systematically starting with the general characteristics of the sample and then becoming increasingly focused on more detailed analysis. Features that may be described include colour, texture and overall particle size. Although very simple parameters, the forensic value of these features is not that significant. Soil colour can vary with moisture content; it can at best be used as a very crude measure allowing soils to be discriminate from one another (e.g. compare a classic red soil from Devon, UK with a clay-rich grey soil from Cornwall, UK). Grain-size analysis is commonly carried out, although it should be noted that there can be differential transfer and retention of different soil/sediment grain size on, for example, different fabrics. Consequently a soil sample collected from an item of clothing may have a different grain size (typically it will be finer grained) than a soil sample collected from a crime scene, even though the soil samples were originally derived from the same place.

Some workers have recommended the analysis of the bulk chemistry of soil samples. However, we would not in general recommend such an approach because most modern analytical approaches (e.g. inductively coupled plasma mass spectroscopy – ICP-MS – appropriate for small sample amounts) require the sample to be dissolved before analysis, hence the geochemical analysis cannot be seen in context with the particles making up that sample. In addition, it is widely recognised that in the analysis of small samples there is a considerable risk of the 'nugget' effect. This is where the inclusion of a small number of particles with a distinctive chemistry may make a sample appear geochemically different to another. Rather than looking at bulk soil/sediment chemistry, in some scenarios the detailed analysis of individual mineral chemistry might be important. There are over a 1000 known mineral types in the United Kingdom; some minerals are very common and occur widely whilst some other minerals only rarely occur, and as such are more typically locality specific. Thus, if such minerals are encountered then their detailed chemical characterisation may be warranted.

The inorganic components present in a soil are naturally occurring minerals along with man-made materials, some of which may themselves have been constructed from geological commodities. Thus, techniques that allow the quantification of a soil's mineralogy are widely used in forensic geoscience. As minerals are typically defined as 'naturally occurring solids with a unique crystalline structure', their identification in most branches of geology typically focuses on techniques that measure characteristic responses related to a mineral's crystal structure. The most common of these is optical microscopy, where polarised light is passed through (or reflected off) a thin cross-section through the sample and the emergent light, which has interacted with the mineral's crystal structure (or lattice), is studied to help in the identification of the mineral (Figure 12.2). However, unless the forensic sample is

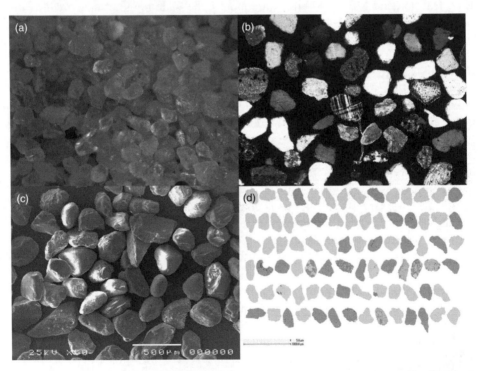

Figure 12.2 There are many different ways in which a soil or sediment sample can be analysed. In this case a sand sample collected from the Omaha D-Day landing beach is imaged: (a) using a binocular microscope, (b) under transmitted light microscopy following the preparation of a sand sample as a thin slice, (c) under manual scanning electron microscopy, and (d) as false colour images of mineral grains identified using automated scanning electron microscopy (QEMSCAN®) analysis; each colour represents a different mineral type. (To see a colour version of this figure, please see Plate 12.2.)

relatively coarse-grained, or if it is a small rock or mineral fragment, then this approach is not usually possible in a forensic context. A more definitive approach is X-ray diffraction. This is where a sample is illuminated with a beam of X-rays and the angle and intensity of the reflections characteristic of the crystal lattice measured. X-ray diffraction (XRD) allows the minerals present to be analysed, although typically if a mineral is present at an abundance of less than 3 % it will not be identified using this approach. In addition, repeated pre-treatments of the sample are required if the detailed clay mineralogy needs to be known.

An alternative approach is the identification of minerals on the basis of chemistry. One major advantage of this approach is that it is relatively simple to map the distribution of elements and therefore to derive a mineralogical image across a sample. Common methods employed include scanning electron microscopy (SEM) with either energy dispersive or wavelength dispersive X-ray spectrometers; or if greater precision is required, the use of electron microprobe analysis. We have utilised automated SEM in the analysis of forensic soil samples in numerous serious crime investigations with considerable success (Figure 12.2), to the extent that peer review scientists (be they working for defence, prosecution, or an outside monitoring agency), will often ask why this method has not been used.

Other techniques that can provide useful information include the examination of the surface texture of sand grains, usually through manual SEM (Figure 12.2). This can be a very useful approach as the surface texture of a sand grain can be indicative of the environment from which that sand grain was derived. In some cases microfossils may be present in a modern soil sample having been derived from the underlying bedrock geology; if present, they can be of considerable evidential value. Thereafter, the nature of the sample and the scene/crime may dictate any specialist analyses. Situations involving engineering failures for instance, may involve analysis of materials by a geologist in conjunction with tests of material strength and durability. Some minerals, microfossils and indeed bone (human and animal) contain characteristic isotopes of elements such as nitrogen, hydrogen, oxygen, carbon and strontium. Measurement of the various isotopes and their ratios can powerfully discriminate minerals in samples and also be used to identify the source of minerals and bone. The latter has been used very successfully in cases of murder victims with no fingerprint or DNA on national databases (see Chapter 7). Isotopic measurements of their teeth, bone, hair and nails can be compared to the global distribution of such isotopes, especially in drinking water, which can direct an enquiry.

12.7 Reporting and court appearance

Because forensic geoscience is not a mainstream forensic tool, it is very important that witness statements and verbal briefings are as clear as possible, and expressed in easily understood language targeted at a non-specialist reader. Clearly technical accuracy must be maintained but the methods adopted and results obtained must be understandable to the investigating team, counsel and ultimately a jury. In most cases a direct 'match' between two samples cannot be demonstrated, unless they were two halves of a broken fragment of rock, which can be perfectly fitted back together. It has been argued that geological trace evidence can only be used to exclude an association between two samples. This is in part because there is no available database on soils which is appropriate for forensic casework. Soils can vary spatially at the metre-scale (and in fact this is why it is a useful class of trace evidence), hence the possibility that there is some other unknown location with exactly the same type of soils as that present at a crime scene cannot be excluded. In general, however, the greater the similarity in characteristics between two samples, the greater the likelihood that they came from the same place. In some cases we have worked on, the suspect's shoes or clothing, or vehicles have different types of soil and mineral dust, the blend of which is only known at one location. Again, it is still possible that another such location exists, but such cases make this associative evidence firmer than the analysis of a single soil type. This likewise applies to using the conjunctive approach we advocate of soil analysis compared to an independent method, for example pollen analysis, or footwear tread. Commonly, though, forensic geoscience statements will be structured such that they are testing the hypothesis that soil sample 1 was derived through contact with exposed soils at locality 2, for example. If the measured characteristics of the soil are very similar, then this is commonly expressed as *'Based on the available data, I cannot exclude the possibility that soil sample 1 was derived through contact with exposed soils at locality 2'*. It is not possible to describe samples as matching; nor is it possible to provide any probabilistic assessment of the similarity between two samples, except for experimental reasons, but certainly not in court. There is still much discussion in the United Kingdom concerning the use of Bayesian statistics in all trace evidence – this is a method of comparing the similarity (or difference) between two samples. The method can be both powerful in simplifying comparison, but does not consider the exclusionary principle, or what chance there is of another such soil occurring in an unsampled alibi location. In general, it is the overall assemblage of particles present which makes a soil distinctive.

Acknowledgements

We thank our colleagues from around the world on the IUGS Initiative on Forensic Geology for sharing their experience and expertise in forensic geology and the various police officers and forensic scientists we have worked with during casework.

References

Murray, R.C. 2004. *Evidence from the Earth: Forensic Geology and Criminal Investigation.* Mountain Press Publishing Company, Missoula, MT.

Pye, K. 2007. *Geological and Soil Evidence: Forensic Applications.* CRC Press, Boca Raton, FL.

Pye, K. and Croft, D.J. (eds) 2004. *Forensic Geoscience: Principles, Techniques and Applications.* Geological Society Special Publication 232, London.

Ritz, K., Dawson, L. and Miller, D. (eds) 2009. *Criminal and Environmental Soil Forensics.* Springer, London.

Ruffell, A. and McKinley, J. 2008. *Geoforensics.* John Wiley & Sons, Ltd, Chichester.

13

Exhibits

Chris Webster
Cheshire Constabulary, Cheshire, UK

13.1   Introduction

The aim of this chapter is to provide forensic practitioners with a good working knowledge of Police Exhibit methodology, thereby equipping them to present their evidence in a manner which is acceptable to the judicial system. For some forensic practitioners and even Police Officers the subject has proved to be needlessly problematic, when perhaps a little knowledge of a few basic principles is all that is required. Hopefully the contents of this chapter will go some way to promoting a better understanding of the subject thereby increasing confidence when collecting and handling exhibits from crime scenes.

Before describing the exhibit methodology in detail it is important to consider why the forensic practitioner needs to know about it at all. Many specialists believe that their role is solely to provide opinion in relation to their particular area of expertise and that the police will take responsibility for the exhibits and documentation surrounding them. In reality, however, the legal system does not differentiate between the police or anyone else involved in gathering evidence. There are certain standards that are expected by the courts and every professional involved in the evidence-gathering process is expected to be aware of and comply with these standards. The consequences of failure to comply with these expectations can range from rendering an element of evidence inadmissible to dismissal of charges, and in the most extreme cases the loss of professional credibility. This is entirely correct given the stakes involved.

It is important to highlight that many of the protocols that have been established in terms of the handling and documentation of exhibits have arisen with the specific aim of avoiding cross-contamination. They have evolved as scientific techniques have become more efficient and as a result of evidence being tested in courts of law.

Interestingly, because of the efficiency of modern scientific recovery techniques, analysis and associated reporting systems, there is often little dispute as to the

Forensic Ecology Handbook: From Crime Scene to Court, First Edition.
Edited by Nicholas Márquez-Grant and Julie Roberts.
© 2012 John Wiley & Sons, Ltd. Published 2012 by John Wiley & Sons, Ltd.

result of scientific examinations. However, within the legal system there are some very good exponents of the 'smokescreen defence' who favour challenging exhibit documentation, packaging and systems, to such an extent that the actual scientific result almost becomes an irrelevant side issue in comparison to the focus and emphasis placed on how forensic practitioners and Police Officers have handled and recorded the exhibits. Consequently, a basic knowledge of exhibit principles is fundamental for all likely to be involved in either recovering or handling exhibits in a professional capacity.

From a practical perspective the two most important maxims to remember when producing exhibits are:

- Keep things simple.

- Always consider how you are finally going to present your evidence to a court or jury in a format that is easy for them to understand.

13.2 Exhibit principles

In order to understand the basic principles involved it is probably useful at this stage to define what an exhibit actually is. It can be defined as '*any object which may have some anticipated evidential value to an investigation*'. If the definition is examined a little more closely, an object can be almost anything with the proviso that it needs to be tangible and have a physical existence. That might sound obvious but in relation to exhibits it has implications in the laboratory as well as at the scene. If an item has been destroyed during a scientific process and it no longer exists, it cannot be exhibited, but in practice this happens fairly infrequently. The practitioner must therefore be familiar with such things as maintaining the integrity and continuity of exhibits and sometimes creating sub-exhibits as part of the examination process.

For the scientific practitioner, objects can range from trace samples at scenes through to body parts and they will usually extend to documents, photographs and other related case material. The qualifying factor which makes an object an exhibit is that it should also have some anticipated evidential value which means that it could possibly be produced to a court or enquiry. Sometimes this creates a dilemma for practitioners who are unsure as to what might be evidential. The rule of thumb here is that if you think an item or sample might be evidential then you should exhibit it from the outset as it can be very difficult to backtrack matters.

It is not the remit of this chapter to explain the rules of disclosure but it is advisable that practitioners acquaint themselves with those rules if they are going to act in a professional capacity as an expert witness. As a minimum they should seek advice from the investigating officers for whom they are acting. Frequently, practitioners gather ancillary material which may help them in their examinations and analyses but which might not ultimately be of evidential value and is therefore unlikely to be produced at court. An example of this might be a historic weather report for a location being investigated, which has been obtained from the Internet. If the data is of value to the practitioner then common sense dictates they may well use it during their investigation. The likelihood is that the police will subsequently obtain direct 'best' evidence from a weather expert as they put their prosecution file together. The original data will not be produced as evidence to the court but should be retained as potential disclosure material by the practitioner. Again, the fallback position is, if in doubt, seek advice from the investigating officers, and treat the item as an exhibit if you think it is going to be produced at court.

Having decided that an item might be of evidential value, it is necessary to consider who produces it and how this is done. Of fundamental importance is that *an exhibit should be produced by the finder.* This sometimes seems to cause headaches for practitioners and again, the maxim is keep things simple. The court's expectation will be that the person producing the exhibit will be able to give some antecedent history in respect of either the item's origin, usage or where it was found.

There has been a growing tendency for Police Officers or Lead Scientists to exhibit all items found at scenes. This is acceptable under certain circumstances providing they can give contemporaneous evidence to the court of where the item was found and how it was created or give some expert contextual evidence. If they cannot fulfil these criteria, then the finder should be the person who can and who actually produces the exhibit.

A common query is, 'What should happen if two or more persons are involved in producing or finding the item?' If this is the case then one of the persons (ideally whoever can give the strongest evidence regarding its history and collection) should produce the item and the other persons involved should then sign the continuity section of the exhibit label and make a witness statement in corroboration.

13.3   Recovery procedures

When it has been decided that an item is an exhibit and who is producing it, the correct procedure must be employed in its recovery. If the following sequence of recovery is undertaken most situations will be adequately catered for:

1. Record initial description, location and, if necessary, scene observations in case notes or logs.

2. Consider record photography *in situ.*

3. Wearing forensic barrier clothing, consider search of the item *in situ* if this is not going to adversely affect the subsequent forensic examination or analysis of it.

4. Package, seal and label the item at the scene.

5. Consider recording any additional relevant detail in notes or logs.

6. Consider changing barrier clothing, certainly gloves or tweezers, if there is a possibility of cross-contaminating any further items within the same scene.

13.4   Labelling exhibits

The first thing that needs to be considered when labelling the exhibit is how to identify the item individually to the practitioner who is producing it. The best way to do
this is for the practitioner to use his or her initials and a sequential number for each
item recovered (Weston, 2002: 30; NPIA, 2005). It is good practice to include middle names as in large-scale enquiries there is a possibility of some people having
the same initials, therefore if John Albert Smith were to produce three exhibits they
would be labelled JAS/1, JAS/2 and JAS/3. Again the advice is to keep it simple.
There has been a tendency within the forensic community to use far more complicated variations of this system, such as JAS/3/01/12/2012/2 representing in this case
Initial/Sequential Exhibit/Date split/Part. Whilst on paper this looks professional it
can be awkward to present in a courtroom environment particularly if there are repeated references to the same exhibit. Thinking ahead to court presentation skills,
how easy is it going to be for a jury to assimilate these long strings of letters and
numbers particularly if there are several that are fairly similar to each other being
repeatedly referred to by an advocate?

If two people have the same initials it is necessary to differentiate between them.
Best practice here is to utilise the second letter of the surname for the second person producing exhibits. Therefore, if John Albert Smith has produced JAS/1 and
Jennifer Angela Swift wishes to produce an exhibit utilising her initials, she should
produce the exhibit as JASW/1.

A lot of modern-day forensic packaging contains an integral exhibit label but if
this is not present, it will be necessary to attach such a label to the packaging you
have used for the item which will be produced. These labels are readily available
either from the police or forensic laboratories. Most of them are of a similar format
containing the headings detailed below:

Identification Ref. No. This is the Exhibit Number. The reference detail of the
person producing in the initial/sequential reference number format previously
explained, that is, JAS/1.

Court Exhibit No. This section is used solely at court. Even if the item has previously been labelled JAS/1, it will be allocated a sequential number by the court
in which it is produced. So if the item was the seventh item produced to a court
during a trial it would be labelled Court Exhibit 7 even though it was produced in a
deposition as JAS/1. The practitioner should therefore leave it blank for court use.

R v. This section is also compiled at court. 'R v' is a shortened version of 'Regina
versus' and the defendant's name will be written in it. Again the practitioner should
leave this section blank.

Description. This is a very important section of the label. Usually a short concise
description is sufficient providing that any additional useful information or extended
description is contained within a statement or log. For example, if a practitioner

had recovered a 'Possible burnt section of fragmented bone' it would be perfectly adequate to describe it as such in the description field of the exhibit label. If it were within the practitioner's expertise and knowledge that they were further able to describe it as '10.5 cm section of possible right femur with head, neck, greater and lesser trochanters intact. Possible hacksaw marks at gluteal tuberosity where bone has been completely severed, lower section not present', then this would of course be useful to both the enquiry and the court and should be fully documented within the scene notes and ultimately the witness statement. The appropriate use of the word 'possible' does give the practitioner a little leeway between recovering the item and being in a position to fully investigate it.

There is no need for overly long descriptions on the label when the appropriate place is within a statement and case file. A title description on the label plus an extended description in case notes and witness statements is both sufficient and practical. A common fault is to also describe the location found within the description field when there is in fact a separate section on the label specifically for this purpose.

Be aware that advocates will expect *an exact replication* of the wording within the description field on any written documentation referring to it, particularly exhibit logs, case notes and witness statements. If there are errors or spelling mistakes within the description field of the label then they should be recorded in exactly the same format in any subsequent records.

Some items can be very difficult to describe fully in written form so consider the use of a sketch or even a photograph when relevant as this can be very useful when trying to present evidence at court.

Time, Date Seized or Produced. This section of the label can provide some interesting opportunities for the exponents of the 'smokescreen defence'. When is an item produced? In the case of an excavated grave for example, is it the time that the practitioner first noticed a possible fragment of bone partially exposed in soil? Is it the time that the bone was excavated and removed? Is it the time that the practitioner completed recording their observations? Or is it the time that the item was sealed in packaging? Obviously the answer could be any of these and in a practical scenario this may well be complicated by the actions and records of CSIs, photographers, or Search Team Officers all carrying out investigation of the scene at the same time and creating their own written notes showing differing times. In practice all would probably be able to agree that they arrived at a site at a particular time, were jointly involved in the recovery process, and able to say that the packaged exhibits were removed at a later time. Under such circumstances it would probably be more realistic to use the same agreed start and finish time for all exhibits (i.e. time of arrival and time of leaving the scene).

There are few circumstances in which individual times would be absolutely necessary. The exception to this might be the recovery of an item with an integral timer that contains data such as a mobile phone or computer or medical samples taken from a victim or deceased person or entomology samples taken with a view to establishing timescales. The key message is that all persons involved in the recovery process should be working to the same recorded times and in practice this means actively seeking confirmation.

Where Seized or Produced. Again, this is a very important section and whereas the description section sometimes contains too much needless detail this section should be completed as fully as possible. Almost certainly, a court and advocates involved in the judicial process will want to know exactly where an item has been found and '123 Acacia Avenue' will not suffice! Within a room or building an exact location is essential, for example 'On top of TV cabinet, room 3 lounge, 123 Acacia Avenue, Anytown'. Keep the description short and concise but ensure it is accurate. The extended description of the location found should be fully documented in both case notes and a witness statement.

Some locations are extremely difficult to describe so there can be huge benefits in drawing additional sketch plans and taking photographs. This can be equally applicable to a range of situations including open land searches (consider using grid systems), storage facilities with multiple shelves and cupboards or multiple pockets within clothing and baggage. Consider using numbers or letters to designate different shelves, cupboards, pockets, etc. or locations within vehicles or buildings. A simple line drawing can be extremely effective and in terms of court presentation the old saying that 'a picture paints a thousand words' is often true. An example of how to designate multiple storage areas is shown in Figure 13.1.

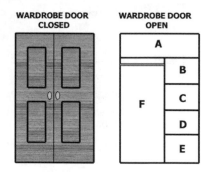

Figure 13.1   Designation of a multiple storage area.

Seized, Produced By. As previously discussed this should be the finder and if more than one person is involved, it should be produced by the person able to give the best evidence and corroborated by persons supporting the find within the continuity section.

Incident/Crime No., Major Incident Item No., Laboratory Ref. These sections are for internal police use and do not require completion by forensic practitioners.

Continuity. Sometimes the continuity section does cause a little confusion for practitioners particularly with regard to how many times they need to sign the exhibit label. *The prosecution has a duty to be able to show strict continuity of all items* *produced in evidence from the time they are seized or produced through to the time they are examined at a scientific laboratory or subsequently produced at court* (ACPO/NPIA, 2006). Currently there are two schools of thought concerning the signing of labels within police circles:

1. Some force policies state that the label should be signed by a witness every time he or she separately handles it. They utilise the label as a method of demonstrating continuity. Clearly for Examining Scientists or Police Exhibit Officers who may be involved in frequent and repeated handling of the same exhibit this can be an onerous task.

2. The alternative, traditional, view is that the label needs only to be signed once, providing the person doing so makes a statement producing the item as an exhibit and refers to any further handling of the item in that or further statements. This method relies on the continuity being recorded in statements and Exhibit Registers. This often used to be supported by an endorsement on many labels which declared 'This is the exhibit referred to in my written statement'. The label also contained endorsements to show compliance with various acts including, 'S9 C.J. Act 1967, s102 M.C. Act 1980 and r 70 M.C. Rules 1981'.

For the forensic practitioner, best practice is to seek early advice from the force they are working with as to what their policy is. If that is not practicable then in the absence of any policy advice, common sense dictates it would be sensible to sign the label on each occasion it changes hands.

A common question posed is 'What should I do if I have forgotten to sign a label?'. It is very important that the signature on the label is not backdated. Simply sign the label with the current date and then compile a statement explaining when the exhibit was actually handled if necessary identifying the exhibit again on the date the label was eventually signed.

Finally, with regard to labelling, it is important not to rely on the label as the sole means of recording an exhibit. Ensure that extended accounts of the information contained within Description field, the Time and Date field and the Where Seized/Produced field are fully documented in both case notes and witness statements describing them. Example of exhibit labels are shown at Figures 13.2, 13.3 and 13.4.

13.5 Key exhibit principles

Both forensic practitioners and the police are expected to comply with certain principles at all times when handling exhibits. Adhering to the principles outlined below will safeguard any evidence obtained.

Integrity. All persons handling exhibits are expected to demonstrate total integrity, namely uprightness, honesty and accountability beyond question. This applies to every aspect of exhibit handling including packaging and documentation.

FORM 123

ANY FORCE CONSTABULARY

Continuity

Identification Ref. No. JAS/1 ...Finder/ Seq No..........

Court Exhibit No. Allocated by the court ....

R -v- Name of defendeant ....

....

Description ....

Short concise title description ....

....

....

....

....

Time/Date Seized/Produced

Parameters may suffice

Where Seized/Produced ....

....

...Full details ....

....

Seized/Produced By

Finder's Name ...Finder's name ....

....

Signed   Signature ....

Incident/Crime No ......Police use ....

Major Incident Item No. Police use ....

Laboratory Ref. .... Police use ....

Name/Rank/No. (Block Capitals)

....

Signed ....

Date ....

Name/Rank/No. (Block Capitals)

....

Signed ....

Date ....

Name/Rank/No. (Block Capitals)

....

Signed ....

Date ....

Name/Rank/No. (Block Capitals)

....

Signed ....

Date.....................................

Name/Rank/No. (Block Capitals)

....

Signed ....

Date.................................... .

Name/Rank/No. (Block Capitals)

....

Signed ....

Date.................................... .

Figure 13.2   Example of an exhibit label.

Preservation. All persons handling exhibits are expected to maintain each exhibit's integrity by ensuring that it is sealed (using signature seals if necessary) and by dealing with it in a manner which demonstrates that nothing has been added to the exhibit or lost from it, either accidentally or deliberately. It should be the aim of the person producing the exhibit to ensure that it is in the state it was originally recovered in, or as near to that as possible, when it arrives at a scientific examination laboratory or is produced at court.

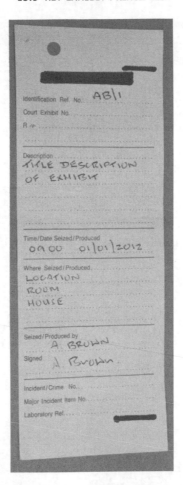

Figure 13.3 Another example of an exhibit label.

In order to do this, it should be sealed at the scene both to preserve it and to prevent any cross-contamination. A lot of modern packaging features integral tamperproof seals, when these are not present then practitioners should consider the use of a signature seal to ensure the exhibit integrity. These types of seals are frequently used with packaging such as paper sacks or knife tubes which do not have manufactured integrity seals. A signature seal is simply a small label containing the handwritten date and signature of the person sealing the item. It is utilised beneath clear sellotape to show who has sealed an item. An example of packaging containing signature seals is shown in Figure 13.4.

Identification. A completed exhibit identification label should be firmly attached to the outside of packaging. The label should be attached at the time the exhibit is produced or seized and signed by all persons handling the exhibit. On larger exhibits it is good practice to write the exhibit reference number on the packaging in addition to the label (Figure 13.5), as this provides a backup should the label become accidentally detached.

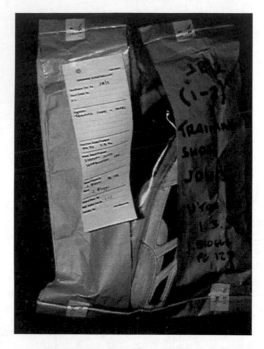

Figure 13.4   Package sealed with signature seal.

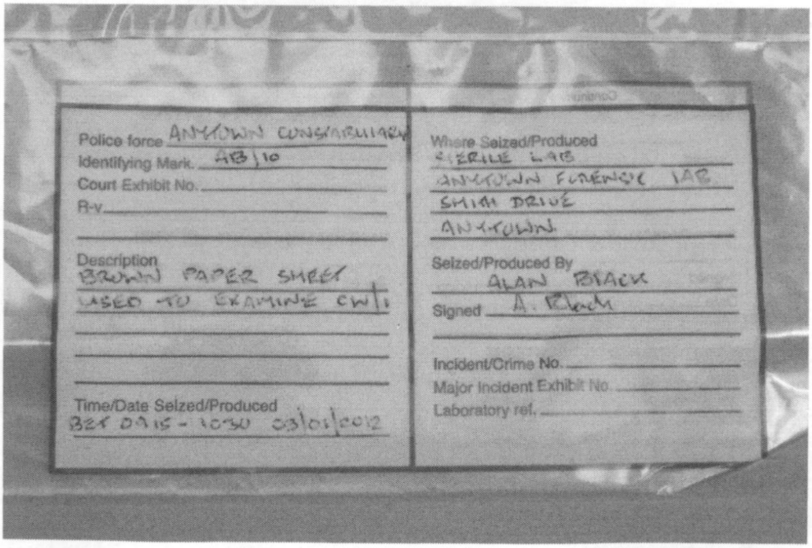

Figure 13.5   Example of information to be completed on an exhibit bag.

Documentation. It is fundamental that the police and their forensic providers are in a position to fully account for all movements of exhibits whilst they are in their control. Normally, the police record such movements in exhibit books, pocket books and investigators' notebooks, transposing the information within them to witness statements. The statement should support corresponding entries on the exhibit labels (NPIA, 2005).

Practitioners should ensure that any movements of exhibits whilst in their possession are properly documented in appropriate case notes or logs and then recorded in witness statements.

13.6 Practical guidelines for exhibit handling

13.6.1 Sealing

Take the packaging to the exhibit and seal it at the scene, not vice versa. This will eliminate the possibility of any cross-contamination and limit allegations of mishandling exhibits. Every time an exhibit is moved both within and outside the scene there is a possibility of cross-contamination. Practitioners should also take care not to take packaging into the scene if it has previously been taken to another scene, as it may well have been contaminated by trace evidence elsewhere.

13.6.2 Labelling

Label the item at the scene, not afterwards. All labels should be completed at the scene and attached there to the sealed packaging. This prevents subsequent errors in identification which could seriously affect the integrity not only of that exhibit but of other evidence presented by the same witness and prosecution. *It would be a reasonable assumption on the part of the court that if a witness has made such an error with labelling then they are likely to have made other errors whilst obtaining other evidence.* Consequently this can have a detrimental effect on that witness' evidence, credibility and integrity.

13.6.3 Description

As previously noted, *keep the description short and concise*, but make sure that it comprises a full and accurate description of what has been recovered. This prevents integrity being reduced by opening packaging, the true benefit of which may only be realised when the exhibit is not accessible to you. In essence, this means that you should obtain a comprehensive description of the item before you seal the exhibit and perhaps transfer it to someone else. If you do not, it may be necessary for you or another person to open the sealed item in order to get that description. This can increase the chances of cross-contamination or allegations of cross-contamination which have the potential to destroy a case or render a piece of evidence unsound. Full descriptions are vital to the police to facilitate their enquiries. This ranges from having sufficient information to interview witnesses and suspects regarding their knowledge of the exhibit to tracing its origin and use in relation to offences being investigated.

13.6.4 Search considerations

A full and thorough search may reveal further items that are of evidential value. The decision to search must be balanced against the necessity to preserve an item for forensic examination. Can sterility be maintained whilst searching? The rule of thumb here is: Can a sterile environment be ensured whilst the item is fully searched, particularly if there is a chance that other trace evidence may be present? Trace evidence might include DNA, fibres, firearms residue, explosives traces, pollen, blood or other body fluids. It is imperative that the correct barrier clothing and mask are worn and if it is felt that the search could be detrimental to these evidence types advice should be sought from the senior scientific advisor at the laboratory or the Senior Police CSM responsible for the scene. There is a balance to be found between preserving the item for all relevant evidence and not finding an urgent item of evidence or intelligence which might well expedite a police investigation. In certain circumstances it may be beneficial to recover and seal an item at a scene and then consider a more detailed search at a properly equipped forensic laboratory.

13.6.5 Sterility

Consider your own environment: is it sterile? The key here is the avoidance of cross-contamination. Are scene suits, masks, gloves and hairnets being worn whilst handling exhibits? Has the correct sequence of dress been observed and is there a need to create a sterile dressing area and sterile exhibit handling area within the scene?

It is important to undertake a through decontamination regime between attending different scenes relating to the same crime and to ensure thorough decontamination between attending other crimes and scenes so that residues or trace evidence are not being transferred into the new scenes. This can equally apply to scientific equipment and packaging material taken from previous scenes to the current scene and it might even include a vehicle or personal clothing which has not even been to a crime scene. An example of this might be socialising at a clay pigeon shoot, or even being in contact with friends who have attended such an event, and then attending a scene at which the police are seeking firearms residue. Before entering the scene it would be imperative to declare to the scene manager your likelihood of contamination.

Defence advocates are very aware of the potential for cross-contamination at scenes and, given the opportunity to do so, they will readily explore the potential of this to discredit evidence

13.6.6 Contamination

To contaminate can be defined as 'To pollute, infect or corrupt' (Thompson, 1996). The importance of avoiding contamination cannot be over-emphasised. Generally, there are four ways in which exhibits are most likely to be contaminated and these are described below.

13.6.6.1 *Contamination prior to packaging*

This may occur due to handling by numerous persons or bags being moved before sealing. Usually, there is no need for more than one person to handle exhibits at a scene. If the item is significant there will be an obvious interest from other parties involved in the investigation but do not pass the item around for second opinions, intelligence gathering, or observation. The potential for cross-contamination here is obvious. As previously described, document the item comprehensively at the scene, consider record photography and sketching, and package it at the scene.

13.6.6.2 *Packaging in contaminated containers*

Ensure the equipment and packaging material used at the scene is forensically sterile and that the material's previous history can be accounted for. Questions to consider include: Has the equipment or material been used or taken to previous scenes? Do you or your organisation have a decontamination regime? If so, where is that policy documented and where are the records of that cleaning regime held, and can they be produced to a court? These are all questions that can legitimately be asked in court and a good forensic practitioner will have prepared in advance so that they can answer these questions if required to do so.

13.6.6.3 *Bags being opened after sealing or never having been sealed originally*

All items should be sealed at the scene at which they are recovered. It is often impossible to immediately rule out the possibility that any exhibit will at some stage in the future have to be scientifically examined to establish if it contains forensic evidence. Good practice is to seal every item in anticipation of this. A further important consideration is that at some stage the police will have to store all the exhibits recovered, *it is imperative that all exhibits coming into their system and stores are sealed* to prevent allegations of cross-contamination.

If an item is properly searched, documented and recorded at the scene with photography if necessary, then this reduces the requirement to open the exhibit to perform any of these tasks. Each time an exhibits package is opened it increases the chance that the item itself could become cross-contaminated again providing fodder for smokescreen defences. The important message here is: record, document search and seal the item at the scene.

13.6.6.4 *Items from different sources being packaged together*

This is perhaps the most common mistake made by both practitioners and Police Officers. Often, out of a desire to save time, items are recovered and exhibited together. There are few cases where this is acceptable. Each individual item has its own forensic story to tell and by placing them together we are altering that information and contaminating it. The primary question to ask here is: What are we trying to preserve and establish? Could the outcome be prejudiced by packaging different items together? If the answer is 'yes' then the items must be packaged separately.

There may be some circumstances when it is acceptable to package some items from the same scene together, but generally this would only be items of the same type. An example of this might be a large number of small shredded and partially burnt fragments of clothing found within a grave or deposition site. Individually, they may not have any identifiable features or relevant trace evidence and the practitioner's objective may simply to be to reconstitute them to try and identify the type or size of clothing to assist an investigation. Under these circumstances the ultimate goal is achievable without prejudicing any forensic recovery.

13.7 Splitting exhibits

A common practical task is the requirement to create new exhibits from within an existing exhibit, this is known as 'splitting' an exhibit or 'sub-exhibiting'. The reasons for this can vary from having to send different parts of the host exhibit to separate laboratories for differing types of examination, to simply identifying a relevant piece of evidence that merits being exhibited separately. As with basic exhibits methodology there is a tendency for both practitioners and Police Officers to over-complicate this process and particularly the documentation surrounding it, including the description. The easiest way to explain this is by practical example below:

> Let us say that CSI John Smith has attended a find of bones located in a water-filled ditch. CSI Smith believes they may be human and recovers the bones to prevent them being lost. On examination CSI Smith logs, photographs, records and exhibits the bones, labelling them:

Quantity of Possible Human Bones   **Ex. Ref. JS/1**

Whilst checking the bones CSI Smith is unsure about the majority of the bones but recognises a bone which within his knowledge and experience he believes is a human right femur and decides to split it from the host exhibit and produce it as a separate exhibit labelling it:

Apparent human right femur – split from quantity of possible human bones JS/1

Ex. Ref. JS/2

Because of the find of the human femur, a forensic anthropologist Anne Marie Davies is tasked to the scene. Anne examines the bones labelled JS/1 and realises that the bones are in fact a combination of animal (non-human) and human bones. Within the content, Anne identifies two further human bones. As Anne is the person who can give an expert opinion and is the author of this evidence, she seizes and produces the two exhibits, labelling them:

Apparent human left ulna – split from quantity of possible human bones JS/1

Ex. Ref. AMD/1

Apparent human mandible – split from quantity of possible human bones JS/1

Ex. Ref. AMD/2

Anne conveys the exhibits back to her forensic laboratory; a further examination takes place, conducted by the senior anthropologist David Joseph Phillips. David conducts various tests and notes the mandible contains a distinctive tooth complete with a filling. Following enquiries with the police a possible victim is identified. As part of the identification process it is decided to show the tooth to the dentist believed to have inserted the filling. To do this David removes the tooth to facilitate the enquiry. David labels the tooth:

Molar tooth – split from apparent human mandible AMD/2

Ex. Ref. DJP/1

Hopefully this narrative explains and demonstrates the methodology involved. The key points are that by labelling the exhibits in this way it is easy to understand where they originated from and how they are connected. In terms of presentation they are labelled in such a way that makes it easy for all parties involved in a court case to follow. The correct methodology has been followed in that the exhibits have been produced by the persons who can give contextual evidence to the court about them. With practice the principle will soon become straightforward.

13.8 Long-term sporadic seizures of exhibits

A frequent dilemma for both practitioners and Police Officers occurs when they are involved in long-term investigations involving the sporadic seizure of exhibits.

Sometimes it may not initially be clear whether scenes are conclusively connected to a particular case, or at the time of attending the scene the specialist or Police Officer is unsure as to how many exhibits they have accumulated at various other scenes in the same particular case. There is clearly a need to produce exhibits at the various scenes but if the witness Andy Brown were to start with Exhibit Reference AB/1 etc. at each scene then there would be confusion and duplicity should the exhibits eventually be produced in the same case or trial. A good practical strategy for this scenario would be as follows:

Should Andy Brown have previously seized approximately 30 exhibits at a scene and then be tasked to another scene, unsure as to exactly how many exhibits he had previously recovered, it would be acceptable for him to commence his exhibits at the second scene with Exhibit Reference AB/101 etc. If Andy were then tasked to a third scene and the same problem occurred, he could commence his exhibits with AB/201 etc. If a fourth scene occurred he could start with AB/301 etc. There may be gaps between the exhibit numbers but these can be explained to the case officers who can document what has happened in the court file. This is a simple and effective solution to this common scenario.

13.9   Unsealing and resealing exhibits for examination

When items are previously recovered and sealed at a scene by Police Officers or forensic practitioners they will usually be submitted for examination at a forensic laboratory. Although forensic laboratories will have their own accredited standard operating procedures in place, some guidelines are given below.

Once the item has been submitted to the forensic laboratories, the forensic practitioner (e.g. forensic examiner) will obviously have to open the bag to access the item for examination. There are a number of practical considerations to this procedure. Firstly, the practitioner should consider whether the item is likely at some later stage to be submitted for examination within another forensic discipline, perhaps DNA or some type of trace work; if so, the item's integrity and continuity will have to be maintained. The forensic practitioner needs to document his or her actions in case notes and perhaps statements. As a precaution, appropriate forensic barrier clothing should be worn. Work surfaces should be sterilised and consideration given to creating an examination area using sterile paper on top of that surface. This can be utilised to capture any fragments of debris or particulates that may be evidential.

To unseal the item a single cut should to be made in the packaging, ideally with a sterile scalpel. It is important that this does not damage the original seals as a court or defence examiners will expect these seals to be preserved intact to show both continuity and integrity. Therefore, the second or subsequent openings should always be completely separate to demonstrate this. Record scale photography is usually a sensible precaution at this stage.

On completion of the examination it is good practice to exhibit the sterile paper sheet separately by folding it on itself – medicine powder style – and sealing it in an appropriate exhibit bag.

The original exhibit bag should be resealed by using two dated signature seals at either end of the cut made into packaging and then securely sealing it with wide clear sellotape (Figure 13.6). The continuity section of the original exhibit label should be signed (Figure 13.7) and any sub- or split-exhibits fully documented. It is not appropriate to return any items after forensic examination unless they have been properly resealed.

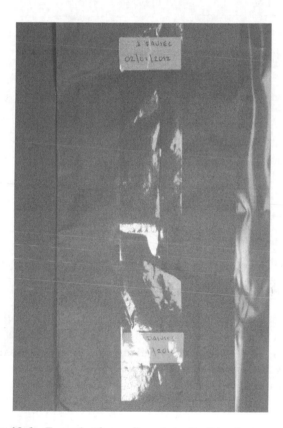

Figure 13.6 Example of re-sealing a bag after it has been cut open.

13.10 Conclusion

Within a single short chapter it is difficult to explore every situation involving exhibits that could potentially arise. An awareness of the basic principles and the practical examples provided should, however, better equip the practitioner to deal with this important aspect of forensic investigation.

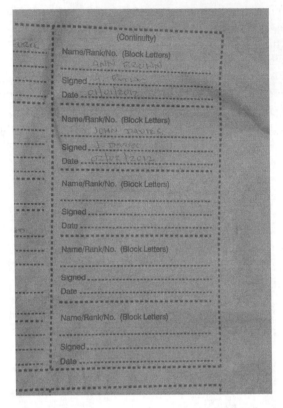

Figure 13.7   It is of utmost importance to sign the continuity information if you have opened a bag.

With practice and experience the practitioner will become more proficient. Remember to have an eye for detail, be methodical and systematic. If you have any queries, consult as soon as practicable with the officers in the case. Finally, remember to keep things as simple as possible with a view to presenting your evidence as effectively as possible at court.

References

ACPO/NPIA. 2006. *Murder Investigation Manual*. ACPO/NPIA, UK.

NPIA. 2005. *Guidance on Major Incident Room Standardised Administrative Procedures (MIRSAP)*. Produced on behalf of the Association of Chief Police Officers, UK.

Thompson, D. (ed.) 1996. *Oxford Compact English Dictionary*. Oxford University Press, Oxford.

Weston, N. 2002. The Crime Scene. In P. White (ed.) *Crime Scene to Court: The Essentials of Forensic Science*. Royal Society of Chemistry, London, pp. 15–46.

14

Forensic photography

John Yoward
Cellmark Forensic Services, Abingdon, UK

14.1   Introduction

Within criminal investigations photography is utilised as a vital investigative tool for many reasons. Images may be taken from a crime scene to present to a court of law to reproduce the scene at the time of the offence. Photography can also be utilised as an evidence-gathering tool for briefing investigative officers, witnesses, or experts involved in the investigation. In order to ensure that evidence gathered and recorded by the civilian expert is sound and admissible in a court of law, it is essential that this is taken and stored in an appropriate manner. Whatever the purpose of the images it is important to remember that a large amount of forensic photography cases will involve the photographer attending a crime scene. It is therefore imperative that the photographer has a thorough understanding of scene discipline in order to preserve forensic evidence as a whole at the scene of crime, and also of best practice guidelines to be adopted during a scene attendance (see Chapter 2). Furthermore, all images taken must be stored and recorded in a particular manner in order to ensure integrity and continuity and enable them to be presented as evidence at court.

This chapter is aimed toward individuals who have a basic knowledge of the theory of photography. It provides further information specific to forensic photography to enable the reader to consider certain issues when recording images at a crime scene in order to produce a crisp and clear image whatever the time of day or night and in whatever challenging environments they may find themselves. This is particularly important when attending the scene of a crime as the photographer will rarely have an opportunity to return for a second chance.

Within forensic photography, knowledge of the technical aspects of the image is vital as the forensic photographer may well be asked in court to provide a technical explanation of an image and must be in a position to provide an answer to any questions put to them.

This chapter emphasises the importance of note-taking and also the methods of recording and storing images that must be adhered to in order to maintain continuity

Forensic Ecology Handbook: From Crime Scene to Court, First Edition.
Edited by Nicholas Márquez-Grant and Julie Roberts.
© 2012 John Wiley & Sons, Ltd. Published 2012 by John Wiley & Sons, Ltd.

and integrity and thus render the material acceptable as evidentially sound for court purposes.

The forensic photographer may also find him or herself in a variety of situations. Two scenarios will be discussed, the mortuary and the outdoor scene.

14.2   Basic elements of photography

We will now take a look at the basic elements of photography, which are key within forensic photography. This section is not intended to teach an individual with no knowledge of photography to be a professional photographer (see Hedgecoe, 2001). It is aimed at individuals who have a basic understanding and knowledge of photography, and will focus on areas that may be worthy of particular consideration both at a crime scene and when recording images within the context of a police investigation.

14.2.1   Exposure

A major factor to be considered in forensic photography specifically is exposure. Getting the exposure right is fundamental. In many situations the camera can do this automatically, but in others the photographer must intervene since there is not always one 'correct 'exposure (Hedgecoe, 2002). The image must be correctly exposed in order to ensure that the subject is clearly identified and any detail contained within it is not restricted by: (a) over-exposure, where too much light is allowed to reach the film/image sensor resulting in bleached out highlight areas; or (b) under-exposure where too little light is allowed to reach the film resulting in loss of shadow detail (McWhinnie, 2000).

An incorrectly exposed image appears unprofessional and may lead to questions from the court as to the photographer's professionalism and perhaps encourage further stringent cross-examination. A further potentially serious issue raised by over- or under-exposed images is that important detail may be lost and could even mislead the court in certain circumstances. Exposure can be measured by either a hand-held meter or, on most modern cameras, an internal meter. In most modern cameras an internal TTL (through the lens) camera meter is viewed when looking into the camera viewfinder. Metering can take various modes, the symbols for each of the commonly used TTL metering modes are shown in Figure 14.1.

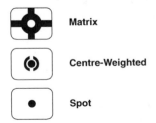

Figure 14.1   Symbols for each of the commonly used TTL metering modes.

- **Matrix metering** is found on most modern single-lens reflex (SLR) and some compact digital cameras. It selects segments of the subject, both highlights and shadow areas, and sets an exposure taking these areas into account, in effect offering an average exposure. This method of metering can be useful for subjects of high contrast in order to obtain an average exposure for the whole scene. This method does, however, have its limitations and is not always suitable for every situation within forensic photography.

- **Centre-weighted metering** will take approximately 70 % of its reading from within the circle shown (Harcourt Davies, 2005). It is therefore in effect a 'middle of the road' system of metering, in-between matrix and spot. Although it is still an option offered by most modern digital SLR cameras it is less commonly utilised by forensic photographers nowadays, but may always be considered.

- **Spot metering** will take its reading from the small area indicated on the screen. It is commonly used within forensic photography for subjects with difficult lighting conditions such as highlights and shadows. It can give the photographer at times more flexibility and control over the exposure, in contrast perhaps to the Matrix meter reading in which the camera is in full control of the whole of the subject. With the spot meter reading the photographer is in control of specific areas, which may be of particular interest to the scene. This mode can also be used at times in order to expose the camera correctly on subjects of extremely low contrast such as markings and minute detail on a white-coloured bone.

After assessing how the camera meter measures the amount of light required to obtain a well-exposed image, the next step is to identify how the camera system controls the amount of light in order to obtain the correct level of exposure to the film/image sensor. This is controlled by two specific functions: the aperture and the shutter speed. In order to understand the direct link between both, Hedgecoe (2002) provides an analogous description of the relationship between the two functions as a cup being filled with water; how long the cup takes to be filled is dependent upon how much the tap is turned on (the lens aperture) and how long the tap is turned on for (the shutter speed).

14.2.2 Aperture

The lens aperture is the opening within a lens, which can be large or small. It is adjustable by the photographer, therefore he or she controls the amount of light that is allowed to fall upon the film/image sensor. The aperture is also commonly known as the *f stop*. It is described on the camera as a number such as *f11*, *f16* or *f22*.

It should be noted that as the aperture becomes smaller the number becomes higher. This can create confusion for some; however it is obtained by dividing the focal length of the lens by the physical size of the whole (aperture). This is known as the relative aperture. The important issue to consider as a photographer is that with every step up the amount of light is halved, for example when the aperture is set at *f4* it will allow twice as much light through to the film/image sensor as when it is set at *f8,* and four times more amount of light as when set at *f16.*

On older cameras, the aperture may be changed by selecting the required number on the lens ring itself. However, on most modern SLR digital cameras both aperture and shutter speed can be changed by making adjustments within the settings of the camera body. It is therefore important for the photographer to become familiar with the equipment they are using.

14.2.3   Shutter speed

In relation to the exposure it is now probably apparent how the aperture and shutter speed are closely linked. The shutter speeds are generally indicated in fractions of a second and apart from the setting B, which may appear on modern SLR cameras, are in a scale which doubles or halves dependent on whether we are travelling up or down the scale. A typical shutter speed scale is shown below:

$$1\,\text{sec} \quad \tfrac{1}{2} \quad \tfrac{1}{4} \quad 1/8 \quad 1/15 \quad 1/30 \quad 1/60 \quad 1/125 \quad 1/250 \quad 1/500 \quad 1/1000$$

Changing the shutter speed from $\tfrac{1}{2}$ second to $\tfrac{1}{4}$ second will clearly halve the amount of light into the lens to fall upon the film/image sensor. However, if the aperture is twice the size, the exposure will be the same and the image will also be correctly exposed. We can now perhaps begin to see where Hedgecoe's (2002) analogy of the tap and running water filling the cup becomes a useful tool for understanding exposure.

The next important factor to consider within forensic photography is the depth of field. Within crime scene photography images are taken to depict the scene accurately for a court, or person who was not there at the time. Therefore in general it is important, when recording a scene digitally, to ensure that the image is as sharp and crisp as possible over the greatest distance possible. This is known as the depth of field. Depth of field can be defined as the distance between the nearest and farthest points of the subject that will appear acceptably sharp on the image (Busselle, Platt and Hilton, 1992). A number of factors affect the depth of field on an image, these factors are listed below:

1. The focal length of a lens. For example, a smaller focal length (18 mm) will have a greater depth of field than a larger focal length lens (210 mm).

2. The camera to subject distance. The depth of field is increased in direct proportion to the camera to subject distance; therefore the further away the subject the greater the depth of field and the closer the subject, the smaller the depth of field.

3. The aperture of the lens. The larger the aperture (smaller the number), the less the depth of field and vice versa.

The depth of field should always be considered by the photographer when they are determining what is required to be depicted in an image. For example, a photograph of a scene showing items of evidence scattered around the area would require a great depth of field to clearly show all the evidence; however, when taking a portrait image of a person a larger aperture may be selected to draw the viewer's attention to the subject and cause a blurring effect to the background behind as seen in Figures 14.2a (at *f22*) and 14.2b (at *f5.6*).

It is important to note that this information is merely an introduction to the subject matter and depth of field can be a complex subject, which requires practice. Some SLR cameras, however, provide an aid and are equipped with a depth of field preview button which allows the photographer to view the depth of field before taking the image. This facility should be utilised on a regular basis by beginners and it is important that photographers are aware of it and are fully conversant with the camera that they are using by reading the manual beforehand.

When selecting which images to take at a crime scene it is important to realise that all images form part of a supplement. The aim of any photographic supplement presented to a court is to tell a story, therefore it is imperative that images are selected carefully to show a particular scene in a logical sequence. Particular methods may be utilised to do this such as the practice of taking a distant view, a mid view and a close-up view.

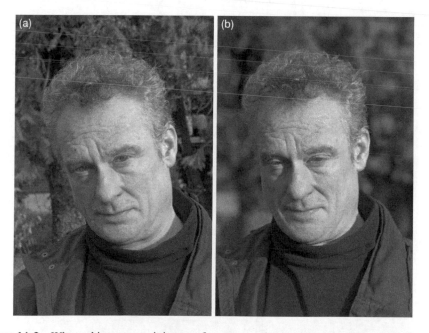

Figure 14.2   When taking a portrait image of a person, selecting a larger aperture will draw the viewer's attention to the subject and cause a blurring effect to the background behind. In image (a) the aperture is set at *f22* and in (b) at *f5.6*. (To see a colour version of this figure, please see Plate 14.2.)

The distant view shows the whole scene. A wide angle lens (18 mm) may be selected and the image should show as much of the scene as is required (Figure 14.3).

The mid view should always be linked to the distant view in some way and the images should be overlapping; in effect assisting the viewer to orientate themselves to the location of the images (Figure 14.4, with a 50 mm lens).

The close view (Figure 14.5, taken with a 200 mm telephoto lens) would generally show a particular area of a scene, paying special attention to detail such as writing on a letter etc.

All three images (Figures 14.3, 14.4 and 14.5) were taken from the same point. However, using different focal lengths of lens, they each have overlapping features. This can tell a story.

Each digital image taken should be recorded along with the number and any other information deemed relevant at the time. It is important to remember that all notes written at the scene and at the time of taking the digital images are disclosable to the court and can be recovered at any time. Therefore, they must be clear, concise and legible enough to be read and understood some period of time later, as on occasions the forensic practitioner or photographer may be asked to describe actions at a scene and explain images in court proceedings some years after the event. Note-taking is crucial.

Items must be recorded before they are moved in any way. At any crime scene items of evidence should only be moved under the direction of the Police CSM or attending CSI. The role of the photographer is to record the scene as it was upon their arrival (see Figure 14.6).

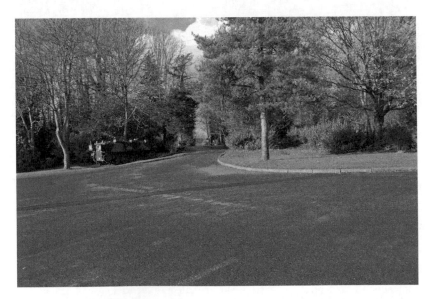

Figure 14.3   Example of a distant view taken with a wide angle lens (18 mm).

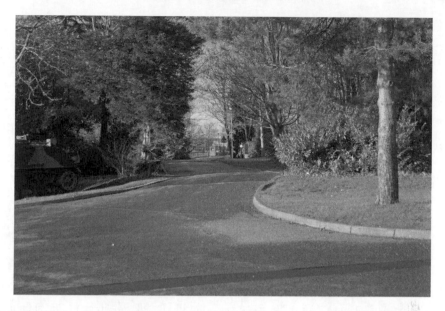

Figure 14.4 A mid view should always be linked to the distant view and the images should be overlapping. The view is taken with a 50 mm lens.

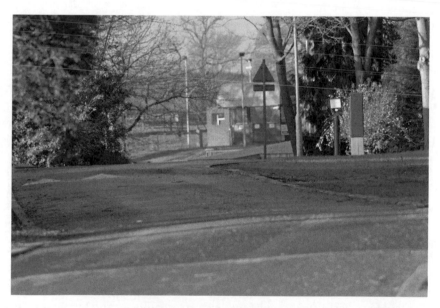

Figure 14.5 A close view of the scene in Figures 14.3 and 14.4, taken with a 200 mm telephoto lens.

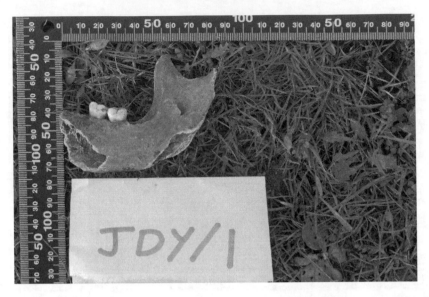

Figure 14.6 Digital images of crime scene items are disclosable to the court and should be recorded as they were on arrival and before they are moved in any way. (To see a colour version of this figure, please see Plate 14.6.)

14.3   Security of images

As a general rule it is better to take too many images as opposed to not enough. However, it must be remembered that all images taken at any potential crime scene are evidential and therefore disclosable. It is therefore imperative that any images taken which are deemed unsuitable remain on the storage media and are not deleted in order to ensure the integrity of the complete set of images. Failure to do this could lead to claims that images which were of great importance had been deleted and could cause considerable issues in judicial proceedings.

Further points to note are that the photographer should always ensure that the media card has been correctly formatted before attending the scene. Simply deleting older images is not sufficient as the numbering system shown on the images will continue to be evidenced, thus potentially allowing the integrity of the images to be questioned when the sequential numbering system does not run consecutively. All cards must be correctly formatted, thereby re-setting the number sequence of the images so there is transparency as to the images taken. Each image recorded at a scene whether used for court purposes or not must be evidenced. Do not be afraid to make mistakes; courts will accept genuine errors by photographers generally without question. However, if it is believed that an attempt has been made to cover up those errors by deleting images, then the issue of integrity and honesty is brought into question, a very serious subject of paramount importance for everybody involved within the criminal justice system.

Once the images have been taken they should be stored as soon as possible on a CD or similar storage device. They should be stored within a WORM ('write once read many') format (PSDB, 2002). The CD should be copied twice in order to ensure that both a master copy (exhibit) and a working copy are maintained. Details such as the name of the photographer, the subject of the images, and the date and time the images were taken should be recorded on the CD to ensure continuity and integrity (PSDB, 2002). It is important to remember that the master CD could potentially be a police exhibit (see Chapter 13); therefore it should be handled in the same way as any other case exhibit so as to maintain the integrity of that exhibit. It should be signature-sealed immediately after downloading and stored securely by the photographer for production if ever required by a court (PSDB, 2002).

14.4   The forensic photographer and the crime scene

It is important to understand that a crime scene in any major investigation may not only be the place where a body is found. The police must consider lots of potential avenues of enquiry such as where the victim was last seen alive, the place of initial contact between victim and suspect, the attack site, the murder site, the body deposition site, and the vehicle in which the victim's body may have been transported. Each of these locations in any major investigation will be treated as a separate scene of crime by the SIO and each area will be preserved as such (ACPO, 2006). The forensic photographer may be required to attend any of these scenes; however, he or she must always act in accordance with the instructions of the CSM. The photographer will be expected to wear full IPE/PPE (individual/personal protective equipment) in the same way as any other person entering the scene; this may include a Tyvek suit, gloves, mask, overboots and any other protective clothing specific to the hazards as instructed by the CSM. The photographer will also be given a detailed brief on any health and safety issues at the scene, routes to take in and out of the scene and areas not to be touched. Further details of this are contained within Chapter 2.

A full health and safety risk assessment should be carried out by anyone entering the scene. At all times any person present at a crime scene must operate within the terms of the Health and Safety at Work Act 1974 which covers the physical and mental well-being of any individual present whether that person is a police officer or visiting the crime scene in support of the criminal justice system (Pepper, 2005). It is extremely important that anyone visiting a crime scene is aware of this Act and the repercussions of ignoring it, as in extreme circumstances failure to comply with the law may lead to a prosecution of that individual. Due to the very nature of major crime scenes body fluids are likely to be present as well as sharp objects, broken glass, knives, hypodermic syringes, etc. These hazards may not always be visible to the naked eye; therefore all persons attending a crime scene must be alert and extremely observant. It is recommended that anyone entering a crime scene to carry out photography should have prior immunisation against infections such as hepatitis and tetanus. It is also good practice for the photographer to make a note of all equipment taken into the scene ensuring that it is all brought out and none inadvertently left behind.

14.5   The forensic photographer at the mortuary

The same principles apply when the photographer is called to attend the mortuary. Photography within a mortuary environment presents its own unique challenges where health and safety issues require early identification and management. Within the mortuary the photographer must always take instructions and guidance from the mortuary manager or in their absence from the senior person present. All mortuaries will have standing operating procedures and safe systems of work available. It is the responsibility of the individual to read and familiarise themselves with these before taking any photographs.

When working within the mortuary, the photographer must recognise that they are part of a team. This team generally consists of the mortuary staff, the pathologist and police CSI personnel all of whom must work together to carry out the forensic post-mortem process in an efficient professional manner to gather evidence in support of the criminal justice system, and in a manner that preserves the dignity of the deceased person also. Other members of the investigation team may also be present such as the SIO or Deputy SIO, the Exhibits Officer and the Coroners' Officer (ACPO, 2006).

Images are taken within the mortuary for a number of reasons which may include: identification; the photography of scars, birth marks and tattoos; the recording of injuries and injury patterns which may be produced in a court as a record of events. Injuries may also be photographed at the request of the forensic pathologist to incorporate into his or her post-mortem report. These images may be of the exterior of a body such as hypostasis or inside body cavities such as damage to the internal organs.

Furthermore, there may be objects on or in the victim which could be of evidential value such as a ligature and the knot, or the knife still in the body. Whatever the purpose of the image it is important to remember that the images will always have the potential to be evidential therefore must be secured and handled in the same way as any other crime scene image in order to maintain continuity and integrity.

The mortuary environment itself can present many issues for the photographer and the following list should always be adhered to (NPIA, 2008):

- Obtain an initial briefing detailing exactly what is required.

- Store photography equipment in a clean area away from body fluids.

- Do not handle the body – leave this role to the CSI / mortuary staff present.

- Manage backgrounds. It is important when photographing a body that extraneous equipment or individuals are not in the background causing an unnecessary distraction from the subject matter. This may be eliminated by the use of a screen or sheet behind the body.

- Always maintain the dignity of the deceased person. Do not unnecessarily photograph genitalia unless they are specifically required as part of the evidential process to show injury. If possible cover the intimate part with a sheet or other appropriate item.

- Wherever possible use photographic equipment (including scales or rulers) specifically for use within the mortuary in order to prevent contamination. Certain police photographic support departments maintain a mortuary kit which never leaves the mortuary and is only utilised for post-mortem purposes.

14.6   Conclusion

It is apparent that the role of a forensic photographer is varied and challenging and does not only encompass the skills of photography. The forensic photographer also requires other key skills such as forensic awareness, crime scene protocols and evidence-handling skills. This chapter has focused on an overview of some basic photography skills; however, it is not a complete photography study guide nor is it a substitute for a complete photography textbook. 'Practice makes perfect'.

References

ACPO. 2006. *Murder Investigation Manual*. NPIA, UK.

Busselle, M., Platt, R. and Hilton, J. 1992. *The Complete 35 mm Source Book*. Mitchell Beazley, London.

Harcourt Davies, P. 2005. *The Photographer's Practical Handbook*. David & Charles, Newton Abbot.

Hedgecoe, J. 2002. *John Hedgecoe's New Introductory Photography Course*. Mitchell Beazley, London.

McWhinnie, A. 2000. *The Complete Photography Manual*. Carlton Books, London.

NPIA. 2008. Initial CSI Course Notes.

Pepper, I. 2005. *Crime Scene Investigation: Methods and Procedures*. Open University Press, Maidenhead.

PSDB. 2002. *Digital Imaging Procedure*. Home Office, London.

Index

Note: Italicised page numbers indicate that the entry appears in an image or a figure caption.

Forensic Ecology Handbook: From Crime Scene to Court, First Edition.
Edited by Nicholas Márquez-Grant and Julie Roberts.
© 2012 John Wiley & Sons, Ltd. Published 2012 by John Wiley & Sons, Ltd.